£ 1.00

25

nas

Medic

nas

nas

Medical Investigations
A Concise Nursing Text

David R. Thompson SRN, RMN, ONC
Charge Nurse, Coronary Care Unit
Leicester General Hospital

Gerald S. Bowman SRN, RMN
Assistant Director of Nursing Services
Leicester General Hospital

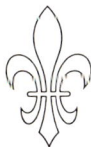

Baillière Tindall London Philadelphia Toronto
Mexico City Rio de Janeiro Sydney Tokyo Hong Kong

| Baillière Tindall | 1 St Anne's Road |
| W. B. Saunders | Eastbourne, East Sussex BN21 3UN, England |

West Washington Square
Philadelphia, PA 19105, USA

1 Goldthorne Avenue
Toronto, Ontario M8Z 5T9, Canada

Apartado 26370—Cedro 512
Mexico 4, DF Mexico

Rua Evaristo da Veiga, 55,20° andar
Rio de Janeiro—RJ, Brazil

ABP Australia Ltd, 44–50 Waterloo Road
North Ryde, NSW 2113, Australia

Ichibancho Central Building, 22–1 Ichibancho
Chiyoda-ku, Tokyo 102, Japan

10/fl, Inter-Continental Plaza, 94 Granville Road
Tsim Sha Tsui East, Kowloon, Hong Kong

© 1985 Baillière Tindall: All rights reserved. No part of this publication
may be reproduced, stored in a retrieval system or transmitted, in any
form or by any means, electronic, mechanical, photocopying or otherwise,
without the prior permission of Baillière Tindall, 1 St Anne's Road,
Eastbourne, East Sussex BN21 3UN, England

First published 1985

Photoset by Paston Press, Norwich
Printed in Great Britain by William Clowes Ltd., Beccles and London

British Library Cataloguing in Publication Data

Thompson, David R.
  Medical investigations.—(NAS)
  1. Nursing
  I. Title II. Bowman, Gerald S. III. Series
  610.73   RT41

ISBN 0 7020 1088 X

Contents

For our children.

Preface

The aim of this small book is to provide the nurse with basic information regarding those common medical investigations that she encounters regularly. It is hoped that the book will be used as an initial reference source in preparing the patient. For this reason each investigation is considered separately, resulting in some inevitable repetition: we make no apologies for this. Although this book is intended primarily for use as a guide to the hospital nurse in the adult care setting, it is anticipated that it may be of value to those nurses who have contact with patients outside the hospital environment.

With this in mind, we have attempted to place this essentially medical subject into the context of nursing care. Although much nursing activity is now self-determined, this is an area where medical delegation is readily accepted. Medical investigations give rise to the need for related nursing care, and we have emphasized the nurse's caring role and the need for close cooperation between nurses and medical staff, which is important in achieving the best outcome for the patient.

It is important for the reader to realize that investigations are only a small part of a whole plan of care; how the nurse understands a particular situation will influence the patient's care. The nurse's responsibility to the patient, notwithstanding her role as the patient's advocate, is paramount. Very often the nurse is the person most likely to understand the patient's reaction towards these investigations. In the text we have given simple explanations of the investigations as a basis for communication with individual patients. The depth of the information given will generally be dictated by the patient's response and the nurse's judgment of circumstances surrounding him. It is hoped that the opening chapters will be useful in providing information related to behaviour that will be likely to result in a successful outcome for the patient.

The text is supported by references and suggestions for further reading. However, the reader should appreciate that although there is a plethora of medical texts related to this subject, there is a paucity of nursing research in this area at the moment and much of the factual nursing advice reflects our own clinical experience.

David R. Thompson   Leicester, 1985
Gerald S. Bowman

1
The Nurse's Role in Investigations: Moral, Ethical, and Legal Considerations

Introduction

Medical investigations are becoming more complicated, rigorous, and precise. Unfortunately, these investigations are very routinized and do not adequately accommodate the patient's individual needs. In order to remedy this neglected area it is important that nurses are aware of certain fundamental issues.

In considering the care of patients undergoing investigations the nurse must take into account any legal, moral, and ethical implications.

The words 'ethics' and 'morals' have similar meanings in the context of behaviour. Ethics is that area of philosophical theory which is concerned with understanding the nature of moral judgments. Morality concerns behaviour which involves judgments, actions, and attitudes based on rationally conceived and effectively established norms.

'Legal' refers to behaviour which is permitted by the law. Nurses are obliged to operate under the umbrella of the civil and criminal law. Very often this umbrella is ill defined: the legal position may be clear on some matters, but uncertain on others.

Codes of ethics

Thompson et al. (1983) point out that 'In practice . . . codes of ethics clearly have their limitations and cannot be seen as always providing the answer to day-to-day moral dilemmas. What such codes can do, however, is to set out the general values and policies in which professional practice is supposed to conform. As such, they provide a means of laying down standards of conduct which a profession might expect its members to meet.' The Royal College of Nursing (1977) notes that such codes are never a substitute for personal moral integrity. The RCN also notes that the nurse's primary responsibility is to protect and enhance the well-being and dignity of each individual in her care. However, nurses also have a responsibility to the profession, to their colleagues, and to themselves.

The substantial growth of interest in ethical problems in nursing is largely due to the scientific and technological advances that have occurred since the second world war, bringing about radical changes in health care. As a result, nurses are starting to question their obligations in clinical practice and to reflect on the morality of their actions.

Patients' rights

The International Council of Nurses' (1973) code of ethics emphasizes fundamental rights and freedoms of individuals—respect for dignity of the individual, and respect for the patient's right to privacy, competent care, and protection from unethical and incompetent practice. Because of the vulnerability and dependence of patients, nurses have in the past often imposed on them their own view of what is best for their welfare. However, nowadays patients have a clearer idea of their rights, and nurses have to be more diligent in making patients feel that their care and well-being are in the hands of competent people. No longer can the nurse pacify the patient with platitudes such as, 'We're doing a little test, but it won't hurt'. This type of approach is an abrogation of moral duty, as every individual has the right to accept or reject what basically amounts to an assault on his body. The nurse's main concern is for her patient. This seems an obvious statement but, in the social system within the health-care setting, consideration of the patient may take second place to that of someone else whom the nurse sees as being more prestigious and wise.

If we accept that the patient has fundamental rights then we, as nurses, have a duty to participate in defending them. This does, however, mean that the nurse must be answerable for any independent action she takes. She is primarily accountable to the patient, but she is also accountable to nurses in higher authority, to her peers, to the profession in general, and to herself. Unfortunately, although nursing claims to be a profession, the hallmarks of autonomy and control over one's own work are difficult to achieve in a bureaucratic framework of management.

The basic rights of the patient are:

1 the right to know;
2 the right to privacy;
3 the right to treatment.

Every patient (or guardian) has the right to be adequately informed about the medical investigation to be performed. He also has the right to privacy, in that he is entitled to respect for his dignity and the confidentiality of information he shares with the nurse and doctor. Every patient has a right to treatment (at least in theory)—a right to expect that he will be cared for and that no harm will occur. However, as Benoliel (1983) points out, 'It is clear that rights are not absolute and that the state can interfere with a person's rights on the basis of the "best interests" of that person or of society.' It must also be appreciated that the patient himself may choose not to exercise his rights.

Confidentiality

The RCN (1980) notes that: 'Confidence is defined . . . as "firm trust"; "in confidence" being defined as a "condition of secrecy".' The responsibility of the nurse regarding confidentiality in law arises from a relationship of trust which exists between the nurse and the patient. In return for sharing information about himself with members of the health care team, the patient is entitled to be told the truth about any medical investigation that is undertaken, particularly in respect of outcome. Patients should have no grounds for fearing that information shared with the staff will be divulged to anyone else, including a relative, without his prior consent. This degree of confidentiality is often overlooked in practice, and more often than not an assumption of consent is made by staff, especially in respect of relatives. Thus, except where required by the law, a nurse should not disclose, without the consent of the patient, information which is obtained in the course of her professional relationship with the patient.

Legal considerations

In an action for damages, a nurse may be held legally liable if it can be shown that she failed to exercise the skills properly expected of her, or that she has undertaken tasks that she was not competent to perform.

Negligence

The nurse must provide the patient with a reasonable standard of care and safety. However, under circumstances of stress, there may have been a breach of that duty. In other words, a negligent act is an act that should not have happened. If a patient is injured or in some way harmed by a careless act, then the nurse may be legally liable to pay compensation, either personally or through an insurance company if the nurse has legal liability insurance. As well as negligent acts or omissions, the nurse can be sued for negligent mis-statements (Young, 1981). Thus the nurse should be careful of the accuracy of the information she gives to patients and relatives.

Consent

It is important that the nurse appreciate the underlying principles of consent. A patient must give consent to enable the nurse, doctor, and other staff to carry out the care needed. If he does not consent, the staff concerned and the health authority may be liable for assault and battery. The patient should only be consenting to that which he clearly understands regarding the actual procedure and its benefits and possible risks. Clearly, therefore, the nurse must ensure that the patient fully understands what is involved. Any queries that she cannot deal with should be referred to the doctor, who has a duty to answer them (Young, 1981). The patient may express consent in a number of ways: he enters hospital voluntarily (except in rare cases), and it may thus be assumed that he is willing to undergo various investigations. He may also express consent by certain actions. Consent can be given verbally, and can be refused verbally. The health authority requires written consent in certain instances legally to ensure that the patient has agreed to undergo certain investigations, e.g. those performed under general anaesthetic.

References

Benoliel, J. Q. (1983) Ethics in nursing practice and education. *Nurs. Outlook* **31**, 210–215.

International Council of Nurses (1973) *Code for nurses: ethical concepts applied to nursing*. Geneva: ICN.

Royal College of Nursing (1977) RCN code of professional conduct: a discussion document. *J. Med. Ethics* **3**, 115–123.

Royal College of Nursing (1980) *Guidelines on confidentiality in nursing.* London: RCN.

Thompson, I. E., Melia, K. M. & Boyd, K. M. (1983) *Nursing Ethics.* Edinburgh: Churchill Livingstone.

Young, A. P. (1981) *Legal Problems in Nursing Practice.* London: Harper & Row.

2
Nursing Care of Patients Undergoing Investigations

Introduction

Rapid scientific and technological advances have made the diagnosis of disease much more refined. As a consequence, the nurse's role in the preparation of patients for diagnostic procedures has become more subtle than giving simple explanations. As Diers (1981) points out: 'Nurses are being expected to help the patient understand what the test means and how the physician or technician will find out something useful from it, as well as give a full explanation of the risks and potential benefits of the procedure'.

Planning the investigation

The hospital setting depersonalizes patients and staff, and the technical and organizational decisions affect the delivery of nursing care. These factors do not help the patient undergoing an investigation, who often feels helpless, anxious, and at times very frightened. Thus it is important that the nurse appreciate those factors which are likely to be helpful and supportive to the patient.

Ideally, investigations should be planned well in advance, with both patient and nurse fully aware of what is intended. Unfortunately, circumstances may dictate that little pre-warning is given about the particular test to be performed, and decisions may be taken in circumstances which provoke anxiety and stress. The patient care area may be busy and noisy, with staff concentrating on the work in hand, resulting in a breakdown in communication between those staff concerned with the test procedure, and between the nurse and patient. Clearly, an effort should be made to focus attention on the patient. Any decisions to be made should be first discussed with the patient and, more importantly, fully understood by him. It should be possible for the patient to visit the area where the test is to take place, and in some instances it may be beneficial for him to see and feel the materials and instruments to be used.

Organization of nursing care

The method of organizing the delivery of nursing care can have a marked effect on whether or not relationships with the patient and his relatives are good, whether the patient feels he is regarded as important, and whether the nurse has the confidence and ability to control or participate in events concerning the patient.

If the system of care is organized around tasks, then it is likely that the nurse's main concern and energies will be directed away from the patient. Alternatively, if the system is organized around the patient (i.e. 'patient allocation'), then close bonding between the nurse and patient should be established, with the nurse more likely to understand the patient's individual needs. A further improvement is the concept of 'primary nursing', whereby qualified nurses have direct nursing responsibility for small groups of patients. In other words, it is the primary nurse who is responsible for assessing the patient's needs after obtaining information about him, identifying his problems, deciding how to tackle them, and evaluating the outcome of the care planned and given. The nurse is placed in a privileged position which encourages in her a feeling of ultimate responsibility for the care of that particular patient.

Information

Providing information to assist the patient's understanding of the procedures to be used is a fundamental function of the nurse. Yet the quality of information given often leaves much to be desired. How many times does one hear a colleague say to a patient: 'Don't worry, we're just going to do a little test'? Do such statements help the patient? It is very doubtful that they do. Do patients understand from the outset the reason why a test is being performed, what it actually entails, how long it will last, whether it will be painful, what the benefits and the risks may be? In fact, are patients given any choice? It is unfortunate but true that patients are rarely given enough verbal information, information booklets, and the results of tests carried out. Yet because the patient does not have accurate knowledge about his condition, and is having to adjust both socially and emotionally to a difficult situation, he needs accurate and comprehensible information to help him.

Information is valuable because it reduces stress, thus giving the patient the ability to control his environment better and enabling him to co-operate and participate in his care (Wilson-Barnett, 1978). Unfortunately, the level of information retained in a stressful situation is not high, and the patient's ability to comprehend and retain information may be further reduced by his anxiety and illness. The nurse must therefore ensure so far as possible that the patient is given relevant information which he can understand and retain.

Wilson-Barnett and Fordham (1982) note that, in medical wards at least, the patient's need for information is most acute prior to investigations. They also cite evidence showing that undergoing diagnostic tests is the most stressful event during a patient's stay in hospital (Wilson-Barnett and Carrigy, 1978), yet few receive information about what will happen.

Although nurses are by nature of their work in a good position to communicate basic information to patients, they rarely do so in a systematic way. Ashworth (1980) highlights the problems nurses have in communicating. Most nurses appear to have had little specific guidance on the amount, content, and methods of communication (verbal and non-verbal). The nurse should ensure that information given about the procedure is based upon individual need. There is something to be gained by asking the patient what he thinks is likely to happen and correcting any misconceptions he may have. The nurse should also appreciate that the patient may wish to ask her certain questions, and be ready to answer them.

Studies such as those of Johnson et al. (1973) and Finesilver (1980) demonstrate that patients need to know what they will experience, for how long, and in whose company. Hartfield et al. (1982) have also demonstrated that patients receiving information about the sensations to be experienced reported significantly less anxiety, and expectations more congruent with their actual experiences, than did subjects receiving information concerned only with the actual procedure. Certainly, a patient will cope more effectively if he is given information prior to a procedure likely to be painful (Hayward, 1975). Hayward's findings also support the contention that 'informed' talking is more effective than 'just talking'.

According to Schuster and Jones (1982), in ideal circumstances nurses would like to spend more time with patients and prepare them better for tests. These investigators found that patients being prepared for barium enema wanted to know the benefits and purpose of the procedure, while nurses believed that this information should be provided by the doctor, not the nurse. Lack of experience and knowledge on the part of the nurse is likely to contribute to the poor quality of information given to patients.

Anderson and Masur (1983) and Wilson-Barnett (1984) provide excellent discussions of the major psychological approaches designed to alleviate patients' concern about procedures, and to enhance their recovery.

It is vital that both medical and nursing staff are in agreement as to what is to happen to the patient and why, and that coherent and consistent information is given to the patient. It does not matter how often information is reiterated to the patient as, under stress, there is a tendency immediately to forget it.

Nurses should always bear in mind that people of different culture, language, intellect, age, or sex, may perceive investigations in different ways. Many patients will feel ignorant, isolated and frightened, dependent on the apparent whim of others. Some will think that no one seems to know what is going to happen, when it will happen, or why. Thus, the onus of responsibility often falls on the nurse to help the patient to understand the nature and purpose of the investigation. Engström (1984) stated that many patients are dissatisfied with the information given as to why investigations are carried out, how to prepare for them, and how the actual investigation will be performed.

It is important to make the initial explanation about a specific investigation simple and direct. The nurse can proceed to further, more detailed, discussion of the procedure according to the patient's level of comprehension.

In conclusion, information will be more effective if it is carefully thought out and planned for each individual patient (Wilson-Barnett, 1979), and if the nurse appreciates the patient's need for and reaction to it.

Reassurance

The main purpose in reassuring patients is to give them the confidence that those caring for them at a time when they are so vulnerable are dependable and supportive. Being dependent on others renders the patient both more vulnerable and less able to make rational judgments for himself (McGilloway, 1976), and he needs to feel that his carers are competent.

French (1979) noted that the phrase 'reassure the patient' frequently occurs in care plans, and made a plea to nurses to avoid using the word 'reassure' because of its ambiguity. In the care plan the nurse should describe exactly the type of behaviour indicated, based on the assessment of the patient's needs. Examples to be considered are: information, familiarization, touch, non-verbal communication, clarification of facts, and encouraging the patient to talk about his fears.

Finally, clichés and platitudes such as: 'Let *us* do the worrying', may satisfy the nurse but are unlikely to do the patient much good.

Nurses' attitudes and opinions

Individual attitudes and opinions are, to a great extent, influenced by the environments and experiences to which a person has been exposed, and patients may be viewed in different ways for a variety of reasons. The nurse is, after all, only human and may not particularly like her patient (Stockwell, 1972). She may, for example, adopt a negative attitude towards a patient who has a history of psychiatric illness (Brady, 1976). Yet such information about a patient should not adversely affect the nurse's attitude towards him. It should be possible for a considerate professional to accept and cope with any limitations a patient may have and still prepare him properly for the investigation. One should be fully aware that the patient's dependency may make him regress emotionally and possibly behave in a totally uncharacteristic manner.

References

Anderson, K. O. & Masur, F. T. (1983) Psychological preparation for invasive medical and dental procedures. *J. Behav. Med.* **6**, 1, 1–40.
Ashworth, P. (1980) *Care to Communicate*. London: RCN.

Brady, M. M. (1976) Nurses' attitudes towards a patient who has a psychiatric history. *J. Adv. Nurs.* **1**, 11–23.

Diers, D. (1981) Clinical and political issues in nursing practice. In: *Current Issues in Nursing.* (Ed. L. Hockey) Edinburgh: Churchill Livingstone.

Engström, B. (1984) The patient's need for information during hospital stay. *Int. J. Nurs. Stud.* **21**, 113–130.

Finesilver, C. (1979) Preparation of adult patients for cardiocatheterization and coronary cineangiography. *Int. J. Nurs. Stud.* **16**, 211–221.

French, H. P. (1979) Reassurance: a nursing skill? *J. Adv. Nurs.* **4**, 627–634.

Hartfield, M. T., Cason, C. L. & Cason, G. J. (1982) Effects of information about a threatening procedure on patients' expectations and emotional distress. *Nurs. Res.* **31**, 202–206.

Hayward, J. C. (1975) *Information: a Prescription against Pain.* London: RCN.

Johnson, J. E., Morrisey, J. F. & Leventhal, H. (1973) Psychological preparation for an endoscopic examination. *Gastroint. Endosc.* **19**, 180–182.

McGilloway, F. A. (1976) Dependency and vulnerability in the nurse/patient situation. *J. Adv. Nurs.* **1**, 229–236.

Schuster, P. & Jones, S. (1982) Preparing the patient for a barium enema: a comparison of nurse and patient opinions. *J. Adv. Nurs.* **7**, 523–527.

Stockwell, F. (1972) *The Unpopular Patient.* London: RCN.

Wilson-Barnett, J. (1978) Patients' emotional responses to barium X-rays. *J. Adv. Nurs.* **3**, 37–48.

Wilson-Barnett, J. (1979) *Stress in Hospital: Patients' Psychological Reactions to Illness and Health Care.* Edinburgh: Churchill Livingstone.

Wilson-Barnett, J. & Carrigy, A. (1978) Factors influencing patients' emotional reactions to hospitalization. *J. Adv. Nurs.* **3**, 221–229.

Wilson-Barnett, J. & Fordham, M. (1982) *Recovery from Illness.* Chichester: Wiley.

Wilson-Barnett, J. (1984) Intervention to alleviate patients' stress: a review. *J. Psychosom. Res.* **28**, 63–72.

3
Investigations Associated with the Gastrointestinal Tract

GASTROINTESTINAL TRACT

The gastrointestinal tract consists of a tube of variable diameter, 9 metres in length, extending from the mouth to the anus. Along its length this complex tube changes in tissue and design so that it can perform its function of ingesting, digesting and absorbing water, electrolytes and nutrients, and excreting unabsorbed food substances and waste products.

Many of the problems that occur in the gastrointestinal tract which require investigation are related to malfunctions such as anorexia, dyspepsia, dysphagia, unexplained vomiting, anaemia, diarrhoea, and constipation.

The gastrointestinal tract is unusual in that it permits relatively easy and direct access for inspection, biopsies and smears, with the use of fibreoptic instruments.

Investigations of this system will be considered in anatomical sequence.

Oesophagus

The oesophagus is a long, hollow, collapsible, muscular tube extending from the pharynx to the cardiac orifice of the stomach. Its function is to transmit food from the mouth through the cardiac sphincter and into the stomach.

The majority of problems encountered in practice tend to occur in the lower third region of the oesophagus; i.e., oesophagitis, oesophageal varices, hiatus hernia, strictures, and occasionally carcinoma.

Stomach

The stomach is the dilated portion of the gastrointestinal tract that lies between the oesophagus and the duodenum. It serves as a reservoir for food and performs the major function of digestion. The stomach extends from the cardiac sphincter to the pyloric sphincter and is essentially J-shaped. Located in the lining of the proximal part of the stomach are the parietal and chief cells which secrete hydrochloric acid (HCl) and pepsinogen respectively. The acid and enzymes mix with the food, beginning the process of digestion. Intrinsic factor, which is essential to the absorption of vitamin B_{12}, is also secreted by the parietal cells. Gastrin is secreted in the mucosa of the distal stomach and, along with the vagus nerve, stimulates HCl and the peristaltic action of the stomach and intestines.

The stomach takes 4–6 hours to empty after a meal.

UPPER GASTROINTESTINAL ENDOSCOPY

This investigation permits direct viewing of the upper gastro-intestinal tract, using a long, flexible, fibreoptic instrument called an endoscope. A camera can be attached to the endoscope, and biopsy forceps or a cytology brush can also be inserted through a channel in the instrument. Suction can be applied to remove secretions and foreign bodies.

Endoscopy is a very convenient and safe method of examining the oesophagus, stomach, and duodenum for tumours, varices, polyps, ulcers and obstructions, hiatal hernias, and mucosal inflammation.

This investigation is performed under a local anaesthetic, usually in the endoscopy clinic by a gastroenterologist. However, the investigation can be carried out at the bedside, in an operating theatre, or in the X-ray department. The procedure takes from 20–30 minutes.

The procedure and its purpose are explained to the patient, who is asked to sign a consent form. The patient should be asked to remove any dentures, jewellery, and clothing from the neck to the waist. It is usually routine for patients to wear a gown, as ordinary clothing may be restrictive and uncomfortable.

It is important that the stomach should be empty prior to this investigation, and a minimum fasting time of 4 hours is usually required. Otherwise it may be necessary to insert a nasogastric tube in order to aspirate the stomach contents.

The gastroenterologist may prescribe a muscle relaxant before the procedure, and this may be given intravenously or orally. A local anaesthetic, in the form of lozenges or spray, may also be given to facilitate easier entry into the oesophagus.

Nursing implications

Most patients are very anxious at the thought of having to swallow a long, apparently thick tube. It is undoubtedly an unpleasant procedure in terms of discomfort, but it is not painful. The patient's anxiety and discomfort may be reduced by careful explanation of such factors as the role of the staff, the equipment to be used, the procedure itself, the sensations to be expected, and the probable outcome (Johnson et al., 1973). The purpose of the investigation should be explained to the patient and relative in simple terms: i.e., 'to look at the lining of the stomach to see if there are any changes and to find out what is causing the discomfort'. The patient should be given time to ask questions and to express his concern or fear; he should not be hurried or his fears brushed aside.

If muscle relaxants or local anaesthetics have been used, their side-effects should be explained to the patient. It is obviously potentially dangerous for him to operate any machinery or drive his car after taking such medication, and he should, therefore, be warned of this in advance, preferably in writing, so that he can make arrangements for the homeward journey if attending as an out-patient.

The patient will require oral hygiene care before and after the test to help ameliorate the discomfort of the procedure. He should also be given the opportunity to empty the bladder before and after the test. Many patients are too embarrassed to ask if they can use the toilet, and they will be unable to speak during the investigations when the endoscope is in position.

After the procedure it is important to check the patient's gag reflex before offering food and fluids: this reflex returns 2–4 hours after the test. The patient should also be given throat lozenges or analgesics to allay any discomfort. The patient should be informed that he may have a sore throat for several days afterwards, and advised to drink cool fluids and gargle with a mouth wash to relieve it.

The nurse should observe the patient for possible complications such as perforation and haemorrhage. Symptoms include epigastric, abdominal, or back pain, dyspnoea, fever, and tachycardia.

Because air is pumped into the stomach to aid inspection of the mucosa, the patient will need to belch and, in many instances, pass flatus, both during and after the procedure. If the patient is told this before the test it may help to reduce his embarrassment.

Patients who have undergone this investigation will have had epigastric symptoms, and the procedure itself may exacerbate existing problems. If so, more careful observation will be required immediately after the procedure.

BARIUM SWALLOW/MEAL AND FOLLOW-THROUGH

This is a relatively simple and usually painless investigation which includes a fluoroscopic and X-ray examination of the oesophagus, stomach, and duodenum. The patient swallows a quantity of barium sulphate (contrast medium) which is observed by means of fluoroscopy and X-ray films as it passes through the gastrointestinal tract.

This investigation is useful for detecting structural abnormalities such as inflammation, ulceration, and tumours of the stomach and duodenum.

The investigation usually involves the introduction of barium into the stomach for a standard barium meal. If double contrast radiography is required, effervescent tablets are given as well, in order to provide a double outline which enables small lesions to be identified. A barium swallow is a modified barium meal, and is used when a lesion of the oesophagus is suspected. A follow-through examination is used to demonstrate the whole of the small bowel, but it is not performed routinely as part of the barium meal.

This investigation is performed in the X-ray department, usually by a radiologist. The barium-meal procedure takes about 20–30 minutes.

The procedure and its purpose are explained to the patient. A minimum fasting time of 6 hours is usually required. If the patient is to have a follow-through examination he should have an aperient on the two nights preceding the examination. The patient should be asked to wear a gown and to remove any necklaces, jewellery, or other item which may show on the X-ray film.

The patient may be asked to take some effervescent tablets which react with the gastric acid, causing a release of gas which provides the double contrast. The patient is then asked to swallow a flavoured barium meal in a calculated amount. The radiologist follows the barium through the oesophagus, stomach, and duodenum using fluoroscopy. X-rays are taken at intervals and in different positions. The positioning is achieved by tilting the X-ray table. If the patient is having the follow-through examination, he will be asked to lie down in a waiting room, and X-rays will then be taken at 30-minute intervals over about 4 hours.

Nursing implications

Most patients find it unpleasant to swallow a relatively large amount of barium emulsion. The nurse should explain to the patient why it is necessary to swallow it, and that a flavour can be added to increase its palatability. The nurse needs to ensure that the patient evacuates the barium, and he should be warned that his stools may be paler in colour because of the barium. He should also be warned of the common complication of constipation, but his normal bowel habits should be ascertained before an aperient or enema is given.

The purpose of the investigation should be explained in simple terms: i.e., 'to look at the lining of the oesophagus (or stomach, etc.) to try and establish the cause of the symptoms'. It should be stressed that although the barium is unpleasant to take, the actual procedure is not too uncomfortable, other than having to lie on a hard table. However, the patient should be warned that the table will be tilted up and down, as this can be alarming if it is unexpected. He should be encouraged to ask questions or express any concerns. Because the investigation may take some time, the patient should be encouraged to bring a book or other material with which to occupy himself.

Once the procedure is over, the nurse should allow the patient the opportunity to rest on a bed if he feels tired. He should be encouraged to eat and drink normally as this will relieve any nausea or indigestion, and it will also encourage expulsion of the barium.

The nurse should observe the patient for any epigastric pain or discomfort. She should tell him to notify the doctor if he has no bowel movement for 2–3 days, as barium can cause faecal impaction.

GASTRIC SECRETION TESTS

The gastric contents are aspirated for analysis to determine the acidity of the stomach in the resting state (basal acid output) and when stimulated by histamine, alcohol, insulin, or pentagastrin (maximal acid output). An increased amount of free hydrochloric acid (HCl) may indicate a peptic ulcer, and an absence of free hydrochloric acid (achlorhydria) may indicate gastric atrophy or pernicious anaemia. The tests are performed for determining the location and type of ulcer, Zollinger–Ellison syndrome, or pernicious anaemia, and for determining the efficacy of treatment.

The Hollander test evaluates the effects of intravenous (IV) insulin on vagus nerve stimulation. Normally, IV insulin causes hypoglycaemia, which increases vagus nerve stimulation and acid secretion. This test is carried out before and after a vagotomy to determine if surgery has been successful: i.e., decreased vagal stimulation and acid secretion.

Histamine or pentagastrin (gastric stimulants) is administered to evaluate gastric cell activity.

The test is performed in a laboratory or on the ward by a nurse or physician. The procedure takes about 3 hours.

The procedure and its purpose are explained to the patient: i.e., 'to find out whether the stomach is secreting too much or too little acid'. The patient should be informed what the test entails, how long it will last, and what he will feel.

The patient should be asked beforehand to stop taking certain drugs, such as anticholinergics, cholinergics, ulcer-healing agents (cimetidine and ranitidine), steroids, antispasmodics and antacids, which may invalidate the test. He should also be asked to avoid alcohol, coffee, and smoking for at least 12 hours before the test.

The patient should be told that a nasogastric tube will be inserted, so that gastric secretions can be aspirated. Also, he will be required to fast 8–12 hours before the test.

Before the test begins, the patient's height and weight should be measured so that the required dose of appropriate gastric stimulant can be calculated. The patient should be informed about these agents and the uncomfortable symptoms that he may experience, including sweating, palpitations, dizziness, and faintness.

During the investigation the patient rests supine on a couch. A nasogastric tube is inserted into the stomach via the nose or mouth, and gastric secretions are aspirated. Specimens are then obtained to evaluate the acidity of the gastric contents and the stimulation test follows. After samples of gastric secretions have been obtained the stimulant is administered, and the gastric contents are aspirated every 15–20 minutes for about 1 hour. During the basal phase an intravenous infusion is set up with a three-way tap connected to the cannula to enable the physician to administer insulin and histamine, if required, and to obtain blood samples.

When the test is complete the nasogastric tube is removed, and the patient is offered a hot drink. Out-patients are advised to have a meal before travelling home. Ideally, a relative or friend should be asked to drive or accompany the patient home.

Nursing implications

Most patients find it unpleasant to have a nasogastric tube inserted into the stomach, so the nurse should explain what is entailed and the necessity for it. She should tell the patient how the nasogastric tube is inserted, i.e., that it is lubricated and passed through the nose or mouth, and that he will be asked to swallow or be given sips of water as the tube is passed into the stomach. The patient's throat may be anaesthetized with a local anaesthetic such as lignocaine.

The patient will be asked to remove any dentures, and will require oral hygiene care before and after the test. He will be more comfortable if he empties his bladder immediately before and after the test.

The nurse should give the patient the opportunity to ask questions and to express any concern or fear. If she cannot adequately deal with them she should refer them to the physician.

The nurse should observe the patient for possible side-effects from the stimulants, such as dizziness, flushing, faintness, headache, tachycardia, and low blood pressure. She should make sure that the appropriate antidote is readily available.

Small intestine

The small intestine is a convoluted tube extending from the pyloric sphincter to its junction with the large intestine at the ileocaecal valve. Anatomically, the small intestine is divided into three segments: duodenum, jejunum, and ileum. Almost all digestion and absorption of food and water occurs in the small intestine. The mucous membrane is special in that it has circular folds which increase the area available for absorption. It also has fine, hair-like projections called villi, and it is supplied with glands which secrete intestinal juice.

Partially digested food (chyme) is expelled through the pyloric sphincter and into the duodenum. At this point the pancreas and biliary tract enter the gastrointestinal tract. The pancreas secretes proteolytic enzymes (trypsin and chymotrypsin), lipolytic enzymes (lipase), and amylatic enzymes (amylase). Digestive enzymes are more suited to an alkaline environment, so water and bicarbonate are also secreted by the pancreas to provide an optimum pH. The biliary system also secretes water and bicarbonate along with bile salts, bilirubin, cholesterol, and phospholipids. In the duodenum the acid chyme stimulates the secretion of cholecystokinin and secretin from the mucosa. These, in turn, stimulate secretions of biliary and pancreatic products of digestion. As the chyme passes through the jejunum and ileum, further digestion and absorption occur.

BIOPSY OF THE SMALL INTESTINE

A specially designed instrument known as a Crosby capsule is used for obtaining a piece of tissue from the small intestine for examination in the laboratory. The Crosby capsule is a small steel cylinder which contains a guillotine mechanism that is activated via a long, thin, flexible, radio-opaque tube.

A biopsy is performed to investigate symptoms of malabsorption; usually coeliac disease. The tissue obtained will indicate the state of the villi and its ability to absorb.

The biopsy is performed by a doctor or a nurse in any setting where the patient can relax. The procedure takes about 2 hours, if all goes to plan. A difficulty may arise when the capsule passes from the stomach into the jejunum.

The procedure and its purpose are explained to the patient, who should have fasted for 4–6 hours beforehand. The patient is asked to swallow the capsule with some water, and the external tube is secured by non-allergenic tape, allowing sufficient length of tube for the capsule to travel through the stomach and duodenum to the jejunum. The patient is asked to lie in the right lateral position so that gravity and the natural contours of the stomach will aid its journey. After an interval of about 1 hour an X-ray is taken of the abdomen and the position of the radio-opaque tube and steel capsule are easily identified.

Once in the correct position the capsule mechanism is ready for activating. A 20-ml syringe charged with clean water is attached to the lumen of the tube, and a small quantity of water is gently syringed down the tube to rid the capsule of any debris. The syringe plunger is then quickly pulled back to draw a small quantity of tissue into the capsule. The suction activates a rubber flange which, in turn, triggers the blade, thus cutting off the piece of tissue that has entered the capsule. The capsule is then slowly withdrawn and the tissue is placed in formalin prior to being transported to the laboratory.

Nursing implications

Most patients are naturally anxious about swallowing the Crosby capsule. However, this anxiety can be allayed by explaining simply that the instrument is smaller in size than many a food bolus. The patient should be informed that the procedure is not painful and that the capsule can be swallowed quite easily with the aid of a drink of water.

The purpose of the investigation should be explained in simple terms: i.e., 'to obtain and examine a piece of tissue from the small intestine'. The patient should be informed that the procedure will not take very long, and that it is quite safe. It will be helpful if the patient can actually see and feel the Crosby capsule beforehand.

It is not unknown for the metal capsule to become detached from the tubing. If this occurs, the patient should be reassured that it will pass naturally out of his body and can be found later in his faeces.

Large intestine (colon)

The large intestine extends from the ileocaecal valve to the anus. It forms an arch which encloses most of the small intestine. The various crude anatomical sites help to describe areas where pathology may present itself; these are the caecum, ascending colon, transverse colon, descending colon, sigmoid colon, and rectum. Water and electrolytes are absorbed in the large intestine, and undigested material (faeces) is moved along into the rectum where it is stored until the time of evacuation.

BARIUM ENEMA

This investigation includes a fluoroscopic and X-ray examination of the large intestine (colon). Barium sulphate (single contrast) or barium sulphate and air (double contrast) is administered slowly through a rectal tube into the colon. The filling process is observed by fluoroscopy, and X-ray films are then taken.

This investigation is useful for detecting the presence of structural abnormalities such as polyps, diverticuli, an intestinal mass, stricture, obstruction, or ulceration.

The investigation is performed in the X-ray department, usually by a radiologist, and takes about 30 minutes.

The procedure and its purpose are explained to the patient, as well as the need for the colon to be cleared of faecal material. The patient will have been on a low-residue diet for 48 hours before the investigation. A cleansing enema should be given the evening before the barium enema. A high colonic washout should be performed 2–4 hours prior to the X-ray examination. Outpatients are usually prepared with diet and oral laxatives, together with suppositories on the morning of the X-ray examination. The patient should be asked to undress completely and to wear a gown.

The patient is asked to lie on the X-ray table in the left lateral position with his knees drawn up. A rectal tube is inserted and barium is slowly administered under fluoroscopy. X-rays are taken at intervals and in different positions. The patient is asked to adopt different positions during the procedure and the table may be tipped backward, so that the barium is moved around the bowel by force of gravity.

Nursing implications

Most patients, especially the elderly, find this investigation uncomfortable and embarrassing. It is therefore exceedingly important to maintain privacy and dignity throughout, and to ensure that the patient feels as comfortable and safe as possible. Informed patients have been shown to be less anxious during X-ray than those who were not given information beforehand (Wilson-Barnett, 1978).

The purpose of the investigation should be explained in simple terms: i.e., 'to attempt to find out the cause of the discomfort (or pain) by putting a substance into the bowel which can be seen on the X-ray film'. The procedure should be explained beforehand in sequence and in simple terms and, ideally, in writing. It is important that the patient is told that it will be uncomfortable (because of the rectal tube and hard table) but not painful. He should be told that this discomfort can be minimized by taking deep breaths through the mouth, which helps to decrease tension and promote relaxation. The importance of adhering to dietary restrictions and bowel preparation should also be stressed. Schuster and Jones (1982) found that nurses believed a patient should have more information than the patients believed they needed, and that patients wanted only minimal detailed information about events that happen *during* the procedure.

Following the procedure, the patient should be encouraged to rest if he so desires. He should be encouraged to eat and drink normally, and should be warned that his stools may be paler in colour because of the barium. The patient should be encouraged to go to the toilet to evacuate the barium and air left in the bowel after the procedure.

The nurse should observe for absence of stools, as retention of barium may cause obstruction and/or faecal impaction. However, she should ascertain the patient's normal bowel habits before intervening.

COLONOSCOPY

This investigation permits direct viewing of the large intestine (colon) by means of a long, flexible, fibreoptic instrument called a colonoscope. Biopsy forceps or a cytology brush can be inserted through a channel of the instrument for obtaining specimens and removing foreign bodies. Polyps can be removed with the use of a snare.

Colonoscopy is performed to examine the colon for the cause of lower intestinal bleeding, diverticular disease, polyps or tumours. It is also performed for diagnosing and evaluating the treatment of ulcerative colitis, and if the results of a barium enema and proctosigmoidoscopy are inconclusive and a lesion is still suspected; or to confirm the findings from these tests.

This investigation is carried out in the outpatient clinic, endoscopy clinic, or X-ray department. The procedure takes from 30 to 60 minutes, depending on the expertise of the operator.

The procedure and its purpose are explained to the patient. All faecal material must be evacuated from the bowel before the examination, and this is usually achieved by careful preparation of the bowel 3 or 5 days beforehand. The 5-day preparation is more likely to achieve better results, but many clinics achieve adequate results with a 3-day preparation.

5-day preparation
A low-residue diet is followed for 5 days prior to the investigation. Twenty-four hours prior to colonoscopy the patient is asked to drink fluids only, and 1 litre of 10% mannitol solution is also given orally. If the patient cannot tolerate mannitol, he is given about 30 ml. of castor oil. On the day of the colonoscopy the patient may still drink clear fluids, and to ensure that the bowel is clear an enema is given.

3-day preparation
Clear fluids are given for 3 full days up to the time of the investigation. Twenty-four hours prior to colonoscopy the patient is given 1 litre of 10% mannitol solution orally. On the day of the colonoscopy an enema is given.

A sedative or tranquillizer may be given orally or intravenously immediately before the investigation to promote relaxation. A few patients may require analgesia, depending on the nature of their condition, which should be considerately assessed prior to colonoscopy.

The patient should be warned that the procedure can cause discomfort, and the staff present should appreciate that he may find the entire proceedings very embarrassing. The patient is asked to lie in the left lateral position with the knees drawn up to the chest. He should be positioned over a disposable sheet, and should be suitably covered to avoid embarrassment and exposure. The colonoscope, warmed and well lubricated, is gently inserted through the anus, its progress up the colon is monitored by fluoroscopy, and X-rays are taken.

Nursing implications

The physical preparation for this investigation is obviously not designed to boost morale, and many patients find it both embarrassing and uncomfortable. The nurse should appreciate this and use her skills to minimize such reactions.

The purpose of the investigation should be explained in simple terms: i.e., 'to attempt to find out the cause of the bowel problem by looking at the lining of the bowel'. The procedure should be explained in simple terms, including bowel preparation, body position, and the time it will take to complete. The patient should be encouraged to relax during the procedure, and to breathe slowly and deeply through the mouth during the insertion of the colonoscope. He should also be informed that he may experience abdominal discomfort if air has been injected into the bowel to improve viewing.

Following the procedure, the patient should be made comfortable and encouraged to rest in bed. He should be warned that anal bleeding may occur, particularly if a biopsy has been taken, but should be reassured that this is expected and will clear up quickly. He should also be told that the air introduced into the bowel during the procedure may cause flatus.

The nurse should observe the patient carefully for possible complications such as haemorrhage and perforation (although these are rare). Symptoms to look for include pain, abdominal distension, and rectal bleeding.

Post-procedure observations will depend on the severity of the presenting symptoms. If this investigation is performed as a routine, the patient should be made aware that air has been pumped into the bowel and he is likely to pass more flatus than normal.

An acutely ill patient, i.e. one with ulcerative colitis, should be closely observed for signs of perforation: i.e., excessive abdominal rigidity and pain.

PROCTOSIGMOIDOSCOPY (PROCTOSCOPY: SIGMOIDOSCOPY)

This investigation permits direct viewing of the anus and rectum (proctoscopy) and sigmoid colon (sigmoidoscopy), using a short (about 7 cm), rigid instrument called a proctoscope, or a longer (about 30 cm), flexible fibreoptic instrument called a sigmoidoscope. Biopsy forceps or a cytology brush can be inserted through a channel in the instrument.

Proctosigmoidoscopy is performed to examine the rectum and the distal sigmoid colon for haemorrhoids, polyps, fistulas, abscess, tumours, ulcers, infection and/or inflammation.

This investigation is performed in the outpatient clinic, on a ward, or in the gastroenterology department, and takes from 15 to 30 minutes.

The procedure and its purpose are explained to the patient. Faecal material must be evacuated before the examination, usually by the administration of an enema or a rectal suppository.

The patient should be warned that the procedure can cause discomfort, particularly if haemorrhoids are present. The patient is asked to lie in the left lateral position with the knees drawn up to the chest. He should be positioned over a disposable sheet, and should be suitably covered to reduce embarrassment and exposure. The proctoscope (or sigmoidoscope), warmed and lubricated, is gently inserted into the rectum.

Nursing implications

Most patients find this investigation embarrassing, and some uncomfortable. It is therefore important that the nurse use good social skills to minimize such effects.

The purpose of the investigation should be explained in simple terms: i.e., 'to find out the cause of the symptoms (bright blood or mucus in the stools) by viewing the lining of the lower bowel'. The procedure should also be explained in simple terms, including bowel preparation, body position, and the time it will take to complete. It is important to tell the patient that the procedure may cause some discomfort, but should not cause severe pain. The patient should be encouraged to breathe deeply and slowly and to try and relax during the procedure. He should also be told there may be abdominal discomfort if air has been injected into the bowel to improve inspection.

Following the procedure, the patient should be made comfortable and encouraged to rest. He should then be encouraged to resume normal activities. If a biopsy has been taken, he should be warned that a small amount of bleeding may occur, but that there is no need for concern.

The nurse should observe the patient for possible complications such as perforation and haemorrhage (although these are rare). Symptoms include pain, abdominal distension, and rectal bleeding. Again, appropriate observation according to the patient's condition should be undertaken.

LIVER, BILIARY TRACT, AND PANCREAS

The liver, biliary tract, and pancreas are often considered together because they are closely related in functions and anatomical sites.

Liver

The liver is the largest organ in the body, occupying most of the right upper quadrant of the abdomen and lying under the diaphragm. Its main functions are: formation and secretion of bile; metabolism and storage of ingested carbohydrates, proteins, and fats; catabolism of endogenous substances such as insulin, gastrin, and steroids; detoxification of drugs and poisons; formation of clotting factors II, VII, IX, and X.

Biliary tract

The biliary tract consists of the gall bladder and the hepatic, cystic, and common bile-ducts. The gall bladder is located under the right lobe of the liver, and its main function is the storage and concentration of bile. The hepatic duct, from the liver, merges with the cystic duct of the gall bladder to form the common bile-duct, which enters the duodenum at the ampulla of Vater.

Pancreas

The pancreas lies close to the stomach and duodenum. Its main functions are endocrine (produce and secrete into the bloodstream glucagon and insulin) and exocrine (produce and secrete digestive enzymes into the gastrointestinal tract via the pancreatic duct). The pancreas also secretes bicarbonate and water in order to neutralize the stomach acid and provide an alkaline environment for digestion.

ENDOSCOPIC RETROGRADE CHOLANGIOPANCREATOGRAPHY (ERCP)

This is an investigation which permits radiographic imaging of the bile-ducts and pancreatic ducts using a long, flexible, side-viewing fibreoptic endoscope. Biopsy forceps and a cytology brush can be attached.

Endoscopic retrograde cholangiopancreatography is a relatively new and safe method for demonstrating obstructing lesions such as stones, benign strictures, cysts, and malignant tumours.

This investigation is performed in either the endoscopy clinic or the X-ray department by a physician or radiologist. The procedure takes about 1 hour.

The procedure and its purpose are explained to the patient, who may be asked to sign a consent form. The patient should be asked to remove any dentures, jewellery and clothing, and to wear a gown before being escorted to the X-ray department where he is asked to lie on a hard table in the left lateral position. The patient is fasted for 6 hours before the investigation. Analgesia, sedation, and a local anaesthetic may be prescribed by the physician. The local anaesthetic may be given to facilitate easier entry of the endoscope into the oral pharynx, to be passed through the oesophagus and stomach and into the duodenum. A fine catheter is passed through the endoscope and introduced into the ampulla of Vater. A radio-opaque dye is then slowly injected under fluoroscopy, and X-ray films are taken.

Nursing implications

Most patients find this procedure very unpleasant. However, anxiety and discomfort can be reduced by careful explanation about the actual procedure, equipment, sensations to be expected, and probable outcome. The patient should be informed that the procedure is not painful but is uncomfortable because of having to lie still on the hard X-ray table, and the initial gag reflex when the endoscope is introduced.

The purpose of the investigation should be explained in simple terms to the patient and relative: i.e., 'to look at the ducts in the pancreas or gall bladder to find out if there is an obstruction'. The patient should be given ample opportunity to ask questions or discuss the procedure in more detail.

If muscle relaxants or local anaesthetics have been used the patient should be advised of the potential hazards. He will require oral hygiene care and possibly throat lozenges to alleviate the resulting throat discomfort. It is also important to check the patient's gag reflex before offering food and fluids after the procedure is over.

The nurse should observe for possible complications such as perforation (which is very painful) although this is rare.

Excessive pain after the procedure may be due to extravasation of the dye into the acini of the pancreas. This pain should be relieved by giving a potent analgesic.

During the procedure air is pumped into the area being examined, and the patient will belch excessively and pass flatus.

LIVER BIOPSY

For this investigation a specially designed needle is inserted through the skin and either through the lower portion of the thorax or through the abdominal wall, and then into the liver. A piece of liver tissue is removed for examination in the laboratory.

Liver biopsy is performed for diagnosing disorders such as cirrhosis, hepatitis, tumours, miliary tuberculosis, amyloidosis, and drug reactions. It is carried out in a clinic or at the patient's bed-side by a physician. The procedure takes about 20 minutes.

Prior to the biopsy, the patient's blood is analyzed for bleeding, clotting, prothrombin times, and platelet counts. The patient's blood is grouped and cross-matched in case haemorrhage occurs.

The procedure and its purpose are explained to the patient, who is asked to undress to the waist and lie, in the supine or left lateral position, on either a bed or a table. The patient is fasted for 6 hours before the procedure, and a mild tranquillizer is given. The skin overlying the area of liver is aseptically prepared and a local anaesthetic is injected into the puncture site. The physician rapidly inserts the biopsy needle into the liver, obtains the tissue, and rapidly withdraws the needle. The puncture site is then dressed, and the patient is asked to lie on his right side to provide pressure on the biopsy site.

Nursing implications

Most patients are very apprehensive about undergoing this procedure, but their apprehension can be allayed if they are given a careful explanation about the procedure, the sensations to be expected, the equipment used, and the probable outcome. The patient should be told that there will be some discomfort, particularly when the biopsy needle is inserted, but that the local anaesthetic will ensure he does not suffer pain.

The purpose of the investigation should be explained in simple terms: i.e., 'to examine a piece of liver tissue to see if it is contributing to his illness'. The patient should be advised to lie very still during the procedure and to hold his breath during exhalation. The patient should be reassured that the procedure is quite safe; complications are markedly reduced when it is performed by an experienced physician.

Once the procedure is completed, the nurse should apply a sterile dressing to the puncture site and explain to the patient why he must lie on his right side. He should be made comfortable, and advised to rest in bed for at least 12 hours.

Most patients experience some shoulder-tip pain when the thoracic route is used. This will respond readily to simple analgesia. The main complication of this investigation is severe haemorrhage. If this occurs in the thorax breathing will be painful and difficult and the blood will have to be aspirated. If the abdominal route has been used the symptoms will be delayed. The blood pressure and pulse rate will indicate haemorrhaging. In both cases, immediate transfusion is essential where excessive haemorrhage has occurred.

References and further reading

Beck, M. L. (1981) Diagnostic tests: 3 common gastrointestinal tests—and how to help your patient through each. *Nursing* **11**, 4, 44–47.

Beck, M. L. (1981) Guiding your patient . . . a step at a time . . . through a colonoscopy. *Nursing* **11**, 6, 28–31.

Bowman, G. S. (1972) Liver biopsy. *Nurs. Times* **68**, 839–840.

Gribble, H. E. (1977) *Gastroenterological Nursing*. London: Baillière Tindall.

Hollanders, D. (1979) *Gastrointestinal Endoscopy*. London: Baillière Tindall.

Johnson, J. E., Morrisey, J. F. & Leventhal, H. (1973) Psychological preparation for an endoscopic examination. *Gastrointest. Endosc.* **19**, 180–182.

Ravenscroft, M. M. & Swan, C. H. J. (1984) *Gastrointestinal Endoscopy and Related Procedures: A Guide for Nurses and Assistants*. London: Chapman and Hall.

Schuster, P. & Jones, S. (1982) Preparing the patient for a barium enema: a comparison of nurse and patient opinions. *J. Adv. Nurs.* **7**, 523–527.

Sykes, M. (1981) *Aspects of Gastroenterology for Nurses*. London: Pitman.

Wilson-Barnett, J. (1978) Patients' emotional reactions to barium X-rays. *J. Adv. Nurs.* **3**, 37–45.

4
Investigations Associated with the Cardiovascular System

CARDIOVASCULAR SYSTEM

The cardiovascular system consists of a pump—the heart—and a network of tubes and blood vessels which enable it to perform its function of providing an adequate blood supply, containing nutrients and oxygen, to the tissues, and removing metabolic waste products from them.

Many of the problems that occur in the cardiovascular system which result in the patient requiring investigation are related to malfunctions causing such problems as pain, breathlessness, palpitations, syncope, and fatigue.

Investigations associated with the cardiovascular system are often perceived as serious and frightening by the patient, so the nurse has an important role in reducing fear by providing adequate information and emotional support.

Heart

The heart is a four-chamber pump composed of two atria and two ventricles. Venous blood returns to the heart via the superior and inferior venae cavae into the right atrium, where it is stored during ventricular systole. During diastole, blood flows from the right atrium across the tricuspid valve into the right ventricle. This ventricle pumps blood across the pulmonary valve into the pulmonary artery, against low resistance. After oxygenation in the lungs the blood returns to the left atrium via four pulmonary veins. The pressure here is considerably higher than in the right atrium. Left atrial blood crosses the mitral valve into the left ventricle, which ejects its contents, against high resistance, over the aortic valve and into the aorta.

ELECTROCARDIOGRAPHY

The electrocardiogram (ECG) is a graphic recording of the electrical activity of the heart as detected on the body surface by electrodes and a galvanometer (ECG machine). This recording can be displayed on moving graph paper or on a screen (monitor) to give a visual impression.

Electrocardiography is an essential part of the examination of the cardiovascular system, but like all investigations must be taken together with all other information. The main clinical value of the ECG is in the interpretation of cardiac arrhythmias, diagnosis of ischaemic heart disease, and in the assessment of ventricular hypertrophy.

The heart possesses certain specialized muscle cells which form the conduction system. This system consists of the sinus node, the atrioventricular junction, which comprises the atrioventricular (A–V) node and the atrioventricular (A–V) bundle, and the ventricular conduction tissue, which comprises right and left bundle branches and peripheral ramifications of the bundle branches.

The sinus node is the normal site of initiation of the heart rhythm. The node is situated at the junction of the superior vena cava with the right atrium. From here the electrical impulse spreads through both atria, causing atrial contraction or depolarization (P-wave of the ECG). The electrical impulse is delayed for approximately 0.04 seconds at the atrioventricular (A–V) node, so that the atria have time to eject their contents into the ventricles and the number of impulses transmitted by the A–V node are regulated. The electrical impulse then travels through the A–V node and A–V bundle, down the bundle branches, and through the terminal ramifications of the ventricular musculature, causing ventricular depolarization (ventricular contraction) (QRS complex of the ECG). The T-wave of the ECG represents ventricular repolarization (ventricular recovery) and is sometimes followed by a small U-wave, the mechanism of which remains uncertain. Repolarization of the atria is often difficult to identify on the ECG because it occurs during the P–R interval and QRS complex. The interval between the end of the QRS complex and the onset of the T-wave is the S–T segment, representing the period of time between depolarization of the ventricles and the period of rapid repolarization. The interval between the P-wave and the QRS complex is the P–R (or P–Q) interval, measured from the onset of atrial depolarization (P) to the onset of ventricular depolarization (Q or R).

The duration of the waves and complexes of the ECG are variable, but the normal durations are:

P–R interval = 0.12–0.20 sec
QRS complex = <0.12 sec

An abnormal ECG indicates a disturbance in the electrical activity of the myocardium.

The ECG is performed at the patient's bedside, usually by a physician, a cardiographer, or an experienced nurse. The procedure takes about 15 minutes.

The procedure and its purpose are explained to the patient. It should be stressed that the ECG machine records the electrical impulses of the heart, but does not send out electric currents, as some patients believe.

It is important that the ECG tracing is not distorted by body movement and electromagnetic interference. For this reason the patient is asked to lie in a supine position, to relax, and remain still and breathe normally during the recording.

It may be necessary to shave excess hair from the chest, so that an adequate tracing can be achieved by the chest electrodes.

Electrodes with pads are strapped to the limbs: right arm (R), left arm (L), and left leg (F). The right-leg electrode is often used to 'earth' the patient. The electrodes are usually in the form of metal plates which are strapped to the wrists and ankles. Electrode jelly is sometimes applied to the plates to ensure good electrical contact with the skin.

Combinations of two electrodes are called bipolar leads: Lead I is the combination of both arm electrodes, Lead II is the combination of the right-arm and left-leg electrodes, and Lead III is the combination of the left-arm and left-leg electrodes. Unipolar leads are AVR, AVL, and AVF (A = augmented, V = voltage, R = right arm, L = left arm, and F = left foot or leg).

Chest leads (or precordial leads) are V_1, V_2, V_3, V_4, V_5, V_6. The standard ECG, therefore, consists of 12 leads; 6 limb leads (I, II, III, AVR, AVL, AVF) and 6 chest (precordial) leads: V_1–V_6.

Chest electrodes are applied to the chest, by suction cups, on specific anatomical sites:

V_1: fourth intercostal space at the right sternal border
V_2: fourth intercostal space at the left sternal border
V_3: midway between V_2 and V_4
V_4: fifth intercostal space in the left midclavicular line
V_5: left anterior axillary line at the level of V_4 horizontally
V_6: left midaxillary line at the level of V_4 horizontally.

Nursing implications

This is an extremely common investigation. It is not unpleasant, it does not cause discomfort, and there are no complications; these points should be stressed to the patient.

The purpose of the investigation should be explained to the patient: i.e., 'to record the activity of the heart'. The procedure should also be explained to the patient with regard to body position, electrode placement, and duration. The patient should be encouraged to relax, remain still, and breathe normally during the recording. He should be asked to avoid tightening the muscles and talking during recording as this may distort the tracing. If he understands this he may not be embarrassed by the subsequent silence during the procedure. If the patient has chest pain during recording, the time of onset should be noted by the nurse.

ECHOCARDIOGRAPHY

This investigation permits imaging of the heart by the use of ultrasound. A probe called a transducer is held over the patient's chest wall to produce an ultrasound beam to the tissues. The reflected sound-waves or echoes from the heart are converted to electrical impulses and recorded on an oscilloscope, moving chart recorder, or videotape.

Echocardiography is a very convenient, safe, and relatively inexpensive investigation. It is particularly popular because it is non-invasive. It can determine the shape, size, and position of the heart and the movement of the heart valves and chambers. The methods commonly used are the M-mode and the two-dimensional mode. The former records the motion of the intra-cardiac structures, and the latter records a cross-sectional view of cardiac structures. The investigation is useful in detecting mitral stenosis, pericardial effusion, congenital heart disease, and chamber enlargement, and in assessing left ventricular function.

This investigation is performed in the echocardiography or X-ray department, by a technician—the echocardiographer, or an experienced cardiologist. The procedure takes about 30 minutes.

The procedure and its purpose are explained to the patient, who is asked to undress to the waist, if able, and then assisted onto the examining table, where he is asked to lie in the supine position. The echocardiographer will apply a special lubricant to the skin surface at the site to be examined, and the transducer is moved by hand across the skin surface.

Nursing implications

Some patients may be anxious when they first see the complicated ultrasound equipment, but their anxiety can be reduced by careful explanation about the staff, equipment, procedure, and duration. The purpose of the investigation should be explained in simple terms: i.e., 'to find out whether the heart is normal in shape and size'. The patient should be given the opportunity to ask questions or express any concern.

The procedure should be explained carefully, the patient being informed that a lubricant will be applied to his chest wall, and that a probe will be gently moved back and forth across the surface. He should be reassured that the investigation is safe and fast, and that he will not be exposed to any hazard such as radiation.

Normal everyday conversation will help the patient to relax before the procedure. However, during the procedure, he should be encouraged to remain still and quiet so that an adequate tracing can be obtained.

CARDIAC CATHETERIZATION

This procedure allows the heart and major blood vessels to be studied. A catheter is inserted into one or more of the heart chambers via a peripheral vein or artery, usually under fluoroscopy. Through the catheter, pressures are recorded, radio-opaque dye is injected for angiography, and measurements of

cardiac output and other cardiac functions are taken. The purpose of the procedure, which is performed under sterile conditions, is: to visualize the heart chambers and vessels by means of
a radio-opaque dye injected into the heart under X-ray control
(angiocardiography or coronary angiography); to measure pressures and record wave-forms from the heart chambers and great
vessels; and to obtain blood samples from the heart for the
measurement of cardiac output and the identification of intra-
cardiac shunting.

Coronary angiography is now the most important and common
of invasive cardiac techniques.

Right heart catheterization:
A radio-opaque catheter is inserted into the femoral vein or an
antecubital vein and advanced through the inferior vena cava,
right atrium, right ventricle, and into the pulmonary artery. The
course is followed by fluoroscopy. Right atrial, right ventricular,
and pulmonary arterial pressures are measured. A radio-opaque
dye is injected and X-ray films are taken. Pressures are recorded
and blood samples are obtained for analysis.

Left heart catheterization:
A radio-opaque catheter is introduced into the brachial or
femoral artery and is advanced into the aorta and then into the
left ventricle (*retrograde aortic technique*). Alternatively, a catheter
is introduced into the *right* atrium using a stilette as a guide. The
trans-septal needle carefully perforates the inter-atrial septum
and the catheter is passed over the needle into the left atrium
(*trans-septal technique*).

Cardiac catheterization is a relatively simple technique, usually requiring only a local anaesthetic and mild sedation for the
patient. The main problem lies in the procedure being invasive.

This investigation is performed in a cardiac catheterization
laboratory or an X-ray department, by a cardiologist, and takes
from 90 minutes to three hours.

The procedure and its purpose are explained to the patient,
who will have been admitted to hospital the day before. The
patient is asked to sign a consent form once the investigation has
been fully explained to him and he has been given the opportunity to express any fears or ask questions.

The day before the investigation, the catheter insertion site will be shaved. Sedation may be prescribed to ensure adequate sleep that night, and the patient is advised that he is to be fasted 4–6 hours before the procedure. Prophylactic antibiotic cover may be prescribed by the physician. Premedication will also be prescribed and given.

The patient is asked to remove any dentures, jewellery, and clothing, and to wear a gown. He is escorted to the department and helped onto the hard table. ECG leads are attached for constant monitoring. The catheter insertion site is aseptically prepared, and the patient is therefore often draped with sterile towels.

Nursing implications

Most patients are very anxious at the thought of undergoing such an investigation. Any apprehension, anxiety, or fear can be allayed by careful explanation about the procedure, equipment, sensations to be expected, staff, and the department where the procedure is to be performed (Finesilver, 1979). The patient should be told what the procedure involves, and it should be stressed that it is not a form of treatment, but a diagnostic and evaluative measure. The patient should be told why it is necessary, how long it will take, the technique used, how the equipment works; and he should be reassured that it is essentially painless, although he may feel some discomfort. The purpose of the investigation should be explained in simple terms to the patient and relative: i.e., 'to see if the arteries of the heart are normal' or 'to check to see if there are any defects in the heart'. The patient should be given ample opportunity to ask questions and to express concern or fear.

The nurse should explain to the patient the sensations he is likely to experience during the procedure: i.e., dizziness as the dye is injected and the table is moved during positioning, palpitations and hot flushes because of the dye. Although transient, the procedure can be uncomfortable. It can also be frightening, especially when the room is darkened during fluoroscopy, and when the staff are all wearing masks and gowns and using complicated-looking equipment. All this must be explained to the patient, who should also be told he will be lying on a hard table for the duration of the procedure, that the room will be darkened at intervals, and that he will be able to ask questions throughout.

If the patient experiences any pain, analgesia should be given immediately to relieve both the pain and the accompanying anxiety.

Once the procedure is completed the incision site is closed by a suture. If the femoral site is used, it is important that pressure be applied for about 15–20 minutes. The wound site is observed for oozing or signs of infection. The extremities are observed for colour, warmth, sensations, and peripheral pulses. Particular attention should be paid to numbness, tingling, or pain. The patient's blood pressure and pulse rate should be recorded at 15-minute intervals.

The patient should be advised to rest in bed, and if he has pain or feels very anxious, narcotic analgesics should be prescribed.

It should be emphasized that coronary angiography is often performed to determine whether a coronary artery bypass graft (CABG) is indicated. Three hundred CABG operations per million population of the UK are needed, according to recent figures (*British Medical Journal*, 1984). With this in mind, the patient should be informed of such a possibility and the likely outcome.

EXERCISE STRESS TESTING (STRESS TESTING; EXERCISE TESTING)

This is an increasingly common investigation that provides valuable information about the heart and circulation. It is based on the theory that patients with ischaemic heart disease (IHD) will have marked ST-segment depression on the ECG when exercising. Depression of the ST-segment and depression or inversion of the T-wave indicate myocardial ischaemia. The ECG, heart rate, and blood pressure are recorded while the patient engages in some form of exercise (stress). The three common methods include climbing stairs, pedalling a stationary bicycle, and walking a treadmill. The aim of the testing is to increase the heart rate to just below maximum levels (i.e., about 160–200 beats per minute in adults). The principle is that coronary arteries that may be occluded will be unable to meet the heart's increased oxygen demand during exercise, resulting in chest pain, fatigue, dyspnoea, excessive tachycardia, or a fall in blood pressure, or the development of life-threatening arrhythmias. If any of these occur, the test is stopped.

On the ECG, ST-segment displacement may occur during or immediately after the test. The test is considered positive when the recording paper shows a depression of the ST-segment of more than 1 mm (0.1 mV) below the baseline. The test is negative when there are no significant ECG abnormalities and the patient experiences no significant symptoms.

Exercise stress testing is becoming more popular because it is non-invasive, is relatively quick and easy to perform, and relatively inexpensive. It is used to confirm a diagnosis of IHD in patients with chest pain; to assess the risk of morbidity and mortality in patients with angina and in survivors of an acute myocardial infarction; to assess the functional capacity of the cardiovascular system; and to evaluate the condition of patients who have participated in cardiac rehabilitation programmes or who have undergone coronary artery bypass surgery.

The investigation is performed in a cardiac investigation laboratory or similar department, by a cardiologist or cardiological technician. The procedure takes from 30 to 45 minutes.

The procedure and its purpose are explained to the patient. The patient is asked to avoid eating, drinking, or smoking for 4 hours before the test. He is asked to undress to the waist and ECG electrodes are placed on his chest and the leads are attached to a monitor. A pre-stress test ECG is then recorded. Blood pressure and pulse rates are also recorded for baseline values.

During testing, the ECG and heart rate (and sometimes blood pressure) are recorded continuously. The test is stopped by the cardiologist if any of the symptoms described occur. After the test, ECG, heart-rate, and blood-pressure recordings are made.

Nursing implications

This is a common investigation which is easily carried out and is not unpleasant or uncomfortable. In fact, many patients appear to find it quite enjoyable. However, some are apprehensive, fearing that it may induce pain or shortness of breath. The nurse needs to reassure these patients that the test will be stopped immediately should such symptoms occur.

The purpose should be explained to the patient: i.e., 'to find out if there is any problem with the blood supply to the heart', or 'to measure the response of the heart to physical stress or exercise'. The procedure should also be explained, emphasizing the need to avoid a heavy meal, or stimulants such as coffee, cigarettes, or alcohol, at least 4 hours beforehand. The patient should also be advised to wear loose, comfortable clothing. He should be asked to avoid wearing slippers as these may cause him to slip—footwear with good grip is much better.

The patient is usually asked to undress to the waist so that ECG electrodes can be applied to the chest, and a blood-pressure cuff to the arm.

The patient should be reassured about safety and comfort and asked to report, during the test, any symptoms of pain, shortness of breath, fatigue, or exhaustion. On completion, the test is stopped gradually, and the patient is asked to continue exercising, but slowly, for about 3 minutes to prevent any sudden change in blood pressure resulting in dizziness.

VECTORCARDIOGRAPHY

The vectorcardiogram (VCG) is a graphic recording of the electrical forces of the heart displayed in the form of a vector loop.

The vectorcardiogram shows a three-dimensional view (frontal, horizontal, and saggital planes) of the heart, whereas the ECG shows a two-dimensional view (frontal and horizontal planes only). Most vectorcardiogram systems use an XYZ lead system. The frontal plane requires the XY combination, the horizontal (transverse) plane requires the XZ combination, and the saggital plane the ZY combination. The resulting vector loop consists of moving, comma-shaped dots which are displayed on the oscilloscope (monitor).

The vectorcardiogram is performed for the diagnosis of myocardial infarction and is useful in the assessment of ventricular hypertrophy. It is carried out in a cardiac laboratory or similar department, by a cardiologist or a technician. The procedure takes about 15 minutes.

The procedure and its purpose are explained to the patient. It should be stressed that it is safe and simple, and is similar to an ECG. The patient should be asked to lie still during recording.

The patient is asked to lie in the supine position. Electrodes are applied, and polaroid films are taken of the vectors displayed on the oscilloscope.

Nursing implications

This is not a common investigation in the UK. However, it is, like the ECG, not unpleasant, it does not cause discomfort, and there are no complications.

The purpose of the investigation should be explained to the patient: i.e., 'to obtain a 3-D recording of the heart'. The procedure should be explained with regard to body position, electrode placement, and duration. The patient should be encouraged to relax, remain still, and breathe normally during recording.

PHONOCARDIOGRAPHY

The phonocardiogram (PCG) is a graphic display of the acoustic events that occur during the cardiac cycle. The phonocardiogram records the heart sounds by the use of a microphone (transducer) placed over the heart. The sounds are electronically detected and amplified and graphically recorded on an oscilloscope (monitor).

The phonocardiogram is used to identify, time, and differentiate various heart sounds and murmurs. It is performed in a cardiac laboratory or similar department, by a cardiologist or a technician. The procedure takes from 15 to 30 minutes.

The procedure and its purpose are explained to the patient. Patients are asked to undress to the waist, if able, and then assisted onto the examining table where they are asked to lie in the supine position. A microphone is placed over various locations on the chest.

Nursing implications

The purpose of the investigation should be explained in simple terms: i.e., 'to listen to and record the heart sounds to see if they are normal'. The procedure, including equipment and duration, should also be explained and the patient told that a lubricant will be applied to the chest wall and a probe placed over various locations on the chest. He should be reassured that the test does not cause discomfort, and is safe and relatively quick.

ARTERIOGRAPHY (ANGIOGRAPHY)

The terms arteriography (examination of the arteries) and angiography (examination of the blood vessels) are interchangeable.

A catheter is inserted into the femoral, brachial, or carotid artery and a radio-opaque dye is injected which, with the aid of fluoroscopy, allows imaging of the blood vessels. The dye may be injected to view the cerebral vessels (cerebral angiography), the pulmonary artery (pulmonary angiography), or the renal artery (renal angiography).

Arteriograms are performed for evaluating blood vessel patency and for identifying abnormal vascularization due to tumours. They are carried out in a cardiac laboratory, X-ray department, or operating theatre, by a radiologist, surgeon, or physician. The procedure takes from 1 to 2 hours.

The procedure and its purpose are explained to the patient, who is then asked to sign a consent form. The catheter insertion site is shaved. The patient is advised to fast for 6 hours before the procedure. Pre-medication, i.e., sedative or narcotic analgesic, is prescribed and given.

The patient is asked to remove any dentures, jewellery, and clothing or any other item which may interfere with viewing, and to wear a gown. He is escorted to the department and helped onto the hard X-ray table, where he is asked to lie in the supine position. The catheter insertion site is aseptically prepared and a local anaesthetic is given.

Nursing implications

Most patients are anxious at the thought of a catheter being inserted and passed into the organ concerned. Such anxiety or apprehension can be allayed by careful explanation about the procedure, equipment, sensations to be expected, staff involved, and the department where the procedure is to be performed. The purpose of the investigation should be explained in simple terms: i.e., 'to look at the blood vessels in the brain (lungs or kidneys) to see if they are normal'. The patient should be allowed to express any concern or fear.

The nurse should explain to the patient the sensations he is likely to experience, i.e., a warm, flushing, or burning sensation when the dye is injected. The patient also needs an explanation about the procedure; i.e., that a doctor will inject a dye into an artery at the groin, elbow, or neck, and the area will be numbed and a catheter will be inserted. It should be stressed that the procedure is not painful, apart from the arterial puncture, but may be uncomfortable at times. He should be informed that he will be lying on a hard table and that photographs will be taken at intervals, including when the room is in darkness, but that he will be able to talk during the procedure, and even look at the films.

Once the procedure is completed, pressure must be applied at the insertion site for about 15-20 minutes. The site is observed for swelling and haematoma. If these occur a cold compress must be applied. The patient's blood pressure and pulse rate should be recorded at 15 minute intervals. Particular attention should be paid to sensations such as numbness, tingling, or pain.

VENOGRAPHY

This investigation is designed to identify and locate thrombi within the venous system of the lower limbs. A radio-opaque dye is injected into the venous system of the affected limb, under fluoroscopy, and X-ray films are taken.

Venograms are performed for the detection of deep vein thrombosis (DVT) and the identification of venous abnormalities. They are carried out in an X-ray department, by a radiologist. The procedure takes from 30 to 90 minutes.

The procedure and its purpose are explained to the patient, who is asked to sign a consent form. No sedation or fasting is usually required, but sedation may be indicated if the patient is extremely apprehensive or is likely to find the procedure painful.

The patient is asked to remove any dentures, jewellery, and clothing, and to wear a gown, before being escorted to the X-ray department and helped onto the hard X-ray table, where he is asked to lie in the supine position. The radiologist injects the dye through a small venous catheter; the course of the dye is followed by fluoroscopy and X-ray films are taken.

Nursing implications

This investigation is not as uncomfortable or as anxiety-provoking as arteriography. The only discomfort is the venous catheterization. The dye may cause a warm, flushing sensation, but it is not as severe as with arteriography. These factors should be taken into consideration when the nurse discusses the investigation with the patient.

The purpose of the investigation should be explained in simple terms, i.e., 'to check for clots in the deep veins of the leg', or 'to check that the deep veins of the leg are functioning normally'. The procedure should also be explained to the patient, including the sensations to be expected, the equipment, including the tilting of the X-ray table, and the intravenous catheter.

Once the procedure is over, the nurse should observe the injection site for bleeding and signs of infection. The patient's blood pressure and pulses should be recorded at 15-minute intervals. The popliteal and femoral pulses should be checked for volume and rate. The nurse should handle the affected limb very gently.

References and further reading

British Medical Journal (1984) Consensus development conference: coronary artery bypass grafting. *Br. Med. J.* **289**, 1527–1529.

Donaldson, R. J. (1981) Sounding out the heart. *Nurs. Mirror* **159**, 6, 40–41.

Finesilver, C. (1979) Preparation of adult patients for cardiac catheterization and coronary cineangiography. *Int. J. Nurs. Stud.* **16**, 211–221.

Hubner, P. (1980) *Nurses' Guide to Cardiac Monitoring.* London: Baillière Tindall.

Thompson, D. R. (1979) Cardiac catheterization. *Nurs. Mirror* **148**, 13, Suppl.

Thompson, D. R. (1982) *Cardiac Nursing.* London: Baillière Tindall.

Thompson, D. R. (1984) Anatomy of the heart. *Nurs. Mirror* **159**, 6, 28–34.

Thompson, D. R. & Anderson, R. H. (1982) Conduction system of the heart. *Nurs. Times* **78**, 310–312.

5
Investigations Associated with the Respiratory System

RESPIRATORY SYSTEM

The respiratory system consists of the nasal passages, pharynx, larynx, trachea, bronchi, and lungs enveloped by the pleura. Air travels through the nose, trachea, bronchus, and bronchioles to end up in the alveoli which, together with their blood supply, form the basic unit of the respiratory system, where the exchange of oxygen and carbon dioxide takes place.

The main problems that occur in the respiratory system which result in the patient requiring investigation are breathlessness, coughing, and pain.

Investigations associated with the respiratory system are often perceived as distressing by the patient, who thinks he will be unable to breathe properly during the procedure.

Lungs

The lungs are elastic structures located in the thoracic cavity. Their outer surface is enveloped by a two-layered protective membrane, the pleura, that covers each lung and lines the thoracic cavity. Between the two layers is a potential space called the pleural space. Each lung is divided into lobes: the right lung has three lobes (upper, middle, and lower) and the left lung has two lobes (upper and lower). Each lobe is divided into segments.

BRONCHOGRAPHY

This investigation involves the introduction of a radio-opaque iodized oil into the bronchi, so that X-ray films can be taken to give a complete outline of each bronchial tree.

The main indication for bronchography is for the detection of bronchiectasis. Although it is often stated that it can be used to detect bronchial obstruction caused by foreign bodies, tumours, or cysts, these are much better seen by bronchoscopy. In fact, the use of bronchography has declined since the advent of fibreoptic bronchoscopy and other modern diagnostic methods such as computed tomography.

Bronchography is performed under a local anaesthetic, or a general anaesthetic, in the X-ray department by a radiologist or chest physician. The procedure takes from 30 to 60 minutes.

The procedure and its purpose are explained to the patient, who is asked to sign a consent form. He will have been required to fast 4–6 hours beforehand. He is asked to remove any dentures, jewellery, or any other material which may be shown on the X-ray film, and to wear a gown.

It is important that the bronchial tree is freed from mucus and secretions, and this is achieved by postural drainage, given for 3 days before the investigation. Potassium iodide, or another expectorant, is also given for 3 days. Potassium iodide is preferred because it indicates whether the patient is sensitive to iodine.

Sedation may be prescribed to promote relaxation, and atropine is prescribed to reduce secretions. These drugs are usually given about 1 hour before the investigation. A local anaesthetic spray is applied to the pharynx and trachea. A catheter is then passed through the nose into the trachea. The catheter is secured in place with non-allergenic tape and the dye is introduced into the catheter. The patient lies supine on the hard X-ray table. During the procedure the patient changes position so that the bronchial tree is filled with contrast dye, under fluoroscopy, and X-ray films are taken.

Nursing implications

Generally, most patients are extremely anxious, and frightened that they may not be able to breathe properly during this investigation. Careful explanation will allay such fears. A well-informed patient is usually relaxed and will contribute to the success of the procedure. Explanation should cover the procedure itself, the equipment, sensations to be expected, duration, staff involved, and probable outcome. It is important to stress that the patient's airway will not be blocked and that he will be able to breathe normally throughout. However, the procedure is not without discomfort and he may have a sore throat after the test due to catheter irritation.

The purpose of the investigation should be explained in simple terms to the patient and relatives: i.e., 'to look at the airways and see if there are any abnormalities'.

The effects, duration, and side-effects of the drugs, in particular the premedication and the local anaesthetic, should be explained to the patient. He should be informed that the drugs will make him feel drowsy and his mouth dry.

The patient will require oral hygiene care before and after the test. He should also be given the opportunity to empty his bladder before and after the test. He should be encouraged to ask questions before the procedure, as he will be unable to speak properly during it.

It is important to check the patient's gag reflex before offering food and fluids after the procedure: this reflex returns 2–4 hours after the test. The patient should also be offered throat lozenges or analgesics for any throat discomfort. He should be encouraged to pay attention to good oral hygiene.

The patient will need to rest in bed afterwards as the procedure is usually exhausting and quite distressing. The nurse should observe the patient's pulse rate and respirations for evidence of respiratory embarrassment.

Extensive physiotherapy may be required to enable the patient to expectorate any remaining dye and secretions.

LUNG ASPIRATION AND BIOPSY

This investigation involves the insertion of a needle through the chest wall and pleura, in order to aspirate or obtain a biopsy for cytology. The main indication is for the diagnosis of a pulmonary tumour, nodule, or acute infection. It is a highly accurate technique in experienced hands.

Lung aspiration and biopsy is performed under a local anaesthetic, in the X-ray department or, more often, on the ward by a physician. The procedure takes about 30 minutes.

The procedure and its purpose are explained to the patient, who is asked to sign a consent form. The patient is asked to undress to the waist and is placed in the recumbent position to reduce the possibility of air embolism. Chest fluoroscopy is usually performed beforehand to determine the most direct route of access. The skin surface area to be punctured is aseptically prepared and a local anaesthetic is injected. If the skin surface is hairy, it may need to be shaved beforehand.

Most patients do not require sedation, but if they are unduly apprehensive it may be necessary in order to achieve the co-operation required in controlling respirations.

A special needle is carefully inserted through the chest wall, and quickly advanced through the pleura during a brief cessation of respiration. This minimizes the risk of causing a pneumothorax due to a tear of the visceral pleura. A syringe is attached to the needle; the needle is rotated and suction is applied to obtain a biopsy. The needle is then quickly withdrawn with the biopsy specimen.

Following the biopsy, the physician usually auscultates the chest, and a chest X-ray is taken to exclude pneumothorax.

Nursing implications

Most patients are anxious and frightened that this may be a painful procedure. A well-informed patient will be more relaxed and cooperative. Explanation should cover the procedure, the equipment, sensations to be expected, duration, staff involved, and probable outcome. It is important to stress that the patient will be able to breathe normally during most of the procedure, and that some discomfort is involved but will be minimized by the local anaesthetic.

The purpose of the investigation should be explained in easy, understandable terms to the patient and relatives: i.e., 'to obtain and examine a piece of lung tissue to see if it is normal'. They should be encouraged to ask questions and informed that sedation may be prescribed by the physician. The effects, duration, and side-effects of the drugs used should also be explained.

It is important that the patient be informed about the need to regulate his breathing pattern during the procedure. He should inform the physician if he wishes to cough and, if he already has a cough, a linctus should be given beforehand.

When the biopsy is completed, the nurse should apply a sterile occlusive dressing to the puncture site. She should ensure that the patient is warm and comfortable, and assess whether he has any discomfort that may require analgesia.

The patient will usually need to rest in bed for about 3 hours afterwards, as he is likely to find the entire procedure distressing and tiring. The nurse should observe his pulse rate and respirations for evidence of respiratory embarrassment, and the wound site for haematoma.

LUNG FUNCTION TESTS

Lung function tests are a method of assessing pulmonary volumes, capacities, and flow rates, by the use of spirometry. The spirometer measures and records various ventilation parameters, including tidal volume (TV), vital capacity (VC), forced expiratory volume (FEV), forced inspiratory volume (FIV), and residual volume (RV).

Vital capacity (VC)

The ability to move air in and out of the chest is measured by recording the volume of air that can be exhaled after a maximum inhalation (vital capacity). The normal adult VC is about 4 litres.

Forced expiratory volume (FEV)

The ability to allow air through the airways depends on their bore: it takes a longer time for a given volume of air to flow through a narrow tube than through a wide tube. Also, there is less air flow in a given time. These two factors are fundamental to the tests for narrowing or obstruction of the airways. The forced expiratory volume in 1 second (FEV_1) is the volume of air exhaled during the first second of the vital capacity. The normal adult FEV_1 is about 3 litres.

One should measure the FEV/VC to obtain the FEV%. In diseases causing obstruction to the airways, the FEV_1 is reduced, and so is the FEV%. Normal people can usually exhale 75% of their vital capacity in the first second. The normal adult FEV% is about 75–80%.

Tidal volume (TV)

This is the volume of air inhaled and exhaled with each normal breath. The normal adult TV is about 500 ml.

Residual volume (RV)

This is the volume of air still remaining in the lungs after a maximal inhalation. The normal adult RV is about 1200 ml.

Total lung capacity (TLC)

This is the total volume of air in the lungs at the end of a maximal inhalation. The TLC can be calculated by adding the vital capacity and the residual volume.

Peak expiratory flow rate (PEFR)

Another method of measuring the volume of air flow in a given time is to record the maximum rate of flow: peak expiratory flow rate. The units of measurement are litres per minute. This is measured with a Wright peak flow meter. The normal measurement range is 400–600 litres per minute. However, this is a maximum *rate* of flow and not the actual volume flowing in 1 minute. The patient is asked to inhale maximally and exhale into the peak flow meter, using a mouthpiece, as fast as he can. The patient is asked to do this on three occasions and the average peak flow rate is recorded.

The values obtained for these tests vary according to factors such as the patient's sex, age, weight, and height.

The main indications for lung function tests are for the evaluation of pulmonary disease and the differentiation between restrictive forms (i.e., pulmonary fibrosis), and obstructive forms (i.e., emphysema, bronchitis, or asthma), preoperative evaluation, and assessment of the effects of treatment (i.e., bronchodilator drugs).

These tests are usually performed in a pulmonary function laboratory or on the ward, by a physician, nurse, technician, or physiotherapist.

Nursing implications

The procedure and its purpose are explained to the patient, who should be free from pain and should have avoided a heavy meal or smoking for 4–6 hours before the tests. If the patient has used any bronchodilators up to 6 hours beforehand, this should be noted. Sedatives and narcotics given before the test may decrease the test results. Medications are not usually restricted unless indicated by the physician. If the patient takes glyceryl trinitrate (GTN) for angina, there should be some available.

The nurse should explain the test in detail to the patient and include information about the procedure, duration, sensations to be expected, outcome, equipment, and staff involved. Above all, she should assure the patient that he will be able to breathe properly. The patient should wear clothing that is comfortable and unrestrictive, such as pyjamas and dressing gown. He should be encouraged to empty his bladder before the tests.

The purpose of the test should be explained simply: i.e., 'to check if the lungs are working normally'. The procedure should be described in sequence, including information about clothing to be worn, avoidance of smoking and heavy meals. There is no need for the patient to remove his dentures.

The patient's age, height, and weight are recorded, and the data is used to predict the normal range. The test is then performed in the sitting or standing position. The patient should be encouraged to practise the breathing pattern required for the test, as he may be apprehensive of the first tests. A nose-clip is applied and the patient is instructed to breathe through the mouth. The patient is usually asked to inhale as deeply as possible and then to exhale as much air as possible.

Occasionally, patients with severe respiratory problems are exhausted after the test and will require planned periods of rest.

The nurse should record the patient's pulse rate and respirations and assess for signs and symptoms of respiratory distress, such as breathlessness, tachycardia, apprehension, and cyanosis.

ARTERIAL BLOOD GAS ANALYSIS

Arterial blood gas analysis gives an indication of the efficiency of the lungs in the exchange of oxygen and carbon dioxide. It usually includes analysis of the arterial pH, partial pressures of oxygen (PO_2) and carbon dioxide (PCO_2), and bicarbonate (HCO_3^-).

This investigation is performed for the assessment of acid-base balance, which may be disturbed due to metabolic or respiratory disorders.

Normal range
pH: 7.35–7.45
PO_2:   80–100 mmHg
PCO_2:   35–45   mmHg
HCO_3:   24–28 mmol/l

If the pH is below 7.35 this indicates acidosis, whereas if it is above 7.45 this indicates alkalosis. The PCO_2 should be measured to determine whether it is a respiratory acidosis which will be indicated by a raised PCO_2 and a low pH.

Arterial blood gas analysis is usually performed on the ward by a physician. The procedure takes about 5 minutes.

The procedure and its purpose are explained to the patient. Arterial blood is usually obtained from the femoral, brachial, or radial arteries. The arterial site is aseptically prepared and a needle, attached to a 2–5 ml syringe containing a small amount of low concentration heparin, is inserted into the artery and the sample of blood is taken.

After the needle is removed, pressure is applied to the puncture site for about 5 minutes to prevent the formation of a haematoma. The syringe is capped and gently rotated to mix the contents and analysis is carried out immediately on a blood gas analyzer machine. Alternatively, the blood sample is placed in a container of ice and immediately taken to the laboratory for analysis.

Nursing implications

The purpose of the procedure is explained to the patient in simple terms: i.e., 'to see if the blood is receiving normal amounts of oxygen'. The procedure should be described in sequence, including the following points. The doctor will be doing the test by taking blood from an artery in the arm or groin, and pressure will be applied to the puncture site for up to 5 minutes to stop bleeding. The patient is usually in the sitting or supine position. The procedure will cause more discomfort than a venous puncture.

If the patient has an abnormal clotting time, or is taking anticoagulant drugs, the nurse should be aware of this as she may need to apply pressure for a longer period. The puncture site is then covered with a sterile dressing.

BRONCHOSCOPY

This investigation permits the direct viewing of the respiratory tract (larynx, trachea, and bronchi) using a fibreoptic instrument called a bronchoscope. This is a flexible tube with a light encased in it to give good illumination. A small channel is connected for suction, and biopsy forceps or a cytology brush can also be inserted through the bronchoscope.

Bronchoscopy is performed to detect a lesion, remove foreign bodies, obtain a biopsy, or to facilitate a free air passage. This investigation is performed under a local anaesthetic, usually in a special department or operating theatre, by a respiratory physician. The procedure takes from 30 to 60 minutes.

The procedure and its purpose are explained to the patient, who is then asked to sign a consent form. The patient is asked to remove any dentures, jewellery, and clothing, and to wear a gown. The patient will have been asked to fast 4–6 hours beforehand.

Premedication, including atropine, is usually prescribed and given about 1 hour before the investigation. The patient's throat is anaesthetized with local spray. The patient is then asked to place himself in the sitting or supine position on the operating table. He is asked to remain still while the bronchoscope is passed down through the mouth or nose.

Nursing implications

Most patients are anxious at the thought of undergoing this procedure. They are particularly worried that they will not be able to breathe properly during the investigation. Careful explanation will help to allay the patient's anxiety and gain his cooperation. Explanation should include information about the actual procedure, equipment, sensations to be expected, duration, outcome, and staff involved. It is important that the patient appreciate that he will be able to breathe during the procedure.

Preparation about breathing during the procedure will depend on the approach the physician will take. If the bronchoscope is to be inserted through the nostril, the patient will be asked to breathe through the mouth. Alternatively, if the bronchoscope is to be inserted through the mouth, the patient should be instructed to practise breathing in and out through the nose with his mouth open. The patient should be told the procedure does cause some discomfort, but that the spray will help to reduce it. He should also be warned that sputum may be bloodstained for a few hours or even days after the investigation if a biopsy has been obtained. He may also have an irritating cough.

The purpose of the investigation should be explained in simple terms to the patient and relatives: i.e., 'to look at the airways to see if they are normal and/or to obtain a specimen'.

The effects, duration, and side-effects of the drugs, in particular the premedication and the local anaesthetic, should be explained to the patient. He should be informed that the drugs will make him feel drowsy and his mouth dry. He should be encouraged to relax before and during the procedure, and the premedication will help.

The patient will require oral hygiene before and after the test. He should be given an opportunity to empty the bladder before and after the test. He should also be encouraged to ask questions before the procedure, as he will be unable to speak properly during it.

It is important to check the patient's gag reflex before offering food and fluids after the procedure: this reflex returns 2–4 hours after the test. The patient should be asked to swallow or cough. He should be told that he may have a hoarse and/or sore throat, and throat lozenges should be offered for mild throat irritation. The importance of good oral hygiene should also be stressed.

If a biopsy has been performed, the patient should be observed for haemoptysis, and his blood pressure and pulse rate recorded.

Although bronchoscopy is usually performed under a local anaesthetic, occasionally a general anaesthetic is required. If this is the case and the patient is unconscious, the nurse should turn him on his side with the head of the bed slightly elevated. The nurse should assess for signs and symptoms of respiratory difficulty: i.e., dyspnoea, wheezing, apprehension, and haemoptysis.

If the patient attends as an outpatient he should be accompanied home by a relative or friend.

References and further reading

Cameron, T. J. (1981) Fibreoptic bronchoscopy. *Am. J. Nurs.*. **81**, 1462–1465.

Duthie, J. (1984) Anatomy and physiology of respiration. *Nursing* **2**, 27, 785–787.

Putman, C. E. Ed. (1981) *Pulmonary Diagnosis: Imaging and other Techniques*. New York: Appleton-Century-Crofts.

Twohig, R. G. (1984) Respiratory function tests. *Nursing* **2**, 27, 807–810.

6
Investigations Associated with the Endocrine System

ENDOCRINE SYSTEM

The endocrine system consists of glands that secrete chemical substances—hormones—which are the main regulators of metabolism, growth and development, reproduction, and the response to stress. Endocrine glands secrete their products directly into the bloodstream, unlike the exocrine glands whose products are secreted through a duct to the site of action. Integration between certain endocrine glands and their target areas, or between endocrine and central nervous mechanisms, is brought about by a series of 'feedback' loops.

The main problems that occur in the endocrine system which result in the patient requiring investigation are due to hyper-secretion or hyposecretion of one or more hormones.

Investigations associated with the endocrine system are usually non-invasive, and although they may be rather distressing, they are not painful.

Thyroid gland

The thyroid gland consists of two lobes connected by a narrow strip of tissue (isthmus). The gland is composed of innumerable small follicles, in the centre of which is thyroglobulin where thyroid hormones are stored. These follicular cells produce triiodothyronine (T_3) and thyroxine (T_4). T_3 is present in small amounts in the blood and is more short-acting and more potent than T_4, the major hormone secreted by the thyroid gland. The ratio of T_4 to T_3 in the serum is at least 25 to 1.

RADIOACTIVE IODINE UPTAKE TEST

This is a useful guide to thyroid function but it is rarely used nowadays. Its purpose is to determine the metabolic activity of the thyroid gland by measuring the absorption of radioactive iodine.

The main indications for a radioactive iodine uptake test are for diagnosing hypo- and hyperthyroidism, for differentiating between hyperthyroidism and an overactive toxic adenoma, and for detecting tumours.

This investigation is performed in a nuclear medicine department by a technician. The procedure takes about 30 minutes.

The procedure and its purpose are explained to the patient who is offered a light breakfast and asked to wear a gown and remove any necklaces.

The patient is escorted to the laboratory and is given a known quantity of radioactive iodine (i.e. ^{131}I or ^{123}I) by mouth (in capsule or liquid form), or alternatively a known quantity of technetium (^{99m}Tc) intravenously. The patient returns to the laboratory at a given time and a scintillation counter is placed over him while he lies on a bed in the supine position. The amount of radioactive iodine (or technetium) accumulated in the thyroid gland is then calculated.

Thyroid scanning with radioactive iodine or technetium is now widely used. A 'hot nodule' is very rarely malignant; 'cold nodules' are usually benign, but have a greater chance of being malignant.

The thyroid gland can also be examined by ultrasound.

Nursing implications

Most patients are not so anxious about the investigation as about the risk of radioactivity. It should be stressed that although the tracer dose has a small amount of radioactivity it is considered harmless. However, women who are pregnant should not be given this test.

The procedure should be carefully explained to the patient, including the equipment used (and its safety), duration, staff involved, and probable outcome. The patient should be informed that the test is not painful, unless an intravenous injection of the radionuclide is given, in which case a little discomfort may be felt.

The purpose of the test should be explained in simple terms: i.e., 'to test the function of the thyroid gland and to find out whether it is acting normally'. The nurse should ascertain whether the patient is allergic to iodine products and assess his intake of large amounts of iodine in food (i.e. fish), drugs, etc.

It is important to inform the patient that the radioactive substance should not harm him or his family, or anyone else, since the dosage is low and gives off very little radiation. He should be introduced to, and made familiar with, the equipment and the noise it makes, and encouraged to talk or ask questions. He should be notified of the times he must return to the laboratory, and told he can eat or drink after about 1 hour.

Pancreas

The pancreas has both endocrine and exocrine functions. The islets of Langerhans are clusters of endocrine secreting cells. The alpha cells secrete glucagon and the beta cells secrete insulin. Insulin's main action is to lower the blood glucose level by facilitating the movement of glucose out of the bloodstream and into the cells of the liver, muscle, or other tissue, where it is used immediately for energy or is stored as glycogen to be used for energy later.

Glucagon tends to raise the blood glucose level by promoting the conversion of glycogen to glucose in the liver. In the absence of insulin, blood glucose levels rise because glucose cannot enter the cells. When the level of glucose exceeds about 180 mg/dl (renal threshold), it spills over into the urine (glycosuria).

ORAL GLUCOSE TOLERANCE TEST

This is still the most specific and sensitive test for confirming the diagnosis of diabetes mellitus. It consists of giving the patient a known amount of oral glucose and obtaining blood and urine samples at regular intervals. It is influenced by a number of factors other than the presence of diabetes; e.g., a previous low carbohydrate intake.

This investigation is performed on the ward by a nurse or physician. The whole procedure takes about 3 hours.

The procedure and its purpose are explained to the patient. Three days before the test, the patient is asked to eat a diet which includes a carbohydrate intake of at least 250 g. Most people normally eat 100–150 g of carbohydrate daily. The patient then fasts from midnight, except for clear fluids, before the test. At a specified time, a blood sample is obtained for a fasting blood sugar, and a urine sample for fasting urine. Then, 50 g of oral glucose dissolved in 200 ml of water is given. The amount may depend on the patient's age and body weight. After the glucose drink has been given, blood and urine specimens are obtained at half-hourly intervals for 2–3 hours, depending on the physician's preference. On completion of the test, the patient is offered a normal diet and is permitted to resume normal activity.

The peak blood glucose level for the oral glucose tolerance test is 30–60 minutes after the ingestion of glucose. The blood glucose level should return to normal in 2–3 hours.

Nursing implications

It is important that patients be given adequate explanation about this test. Written instructions about dietary requirements before the test are essential for optimum compliance.

The procedure should be carefully explained to the patient, including diet, glucose drink, blood and urine samples, duration of test, and probable outcome. The patient should be informed that the test is not painful, apart from the blood sampling. Some units insert a 'Venflon'-type catheter instead of performing repeated venepunctures for obtaining the blood samples.

The purpose of the test should be explained in simple terms: i.e., 'to see if the blood sugar level stays normal'. The nurse should point out that the test determines blood glucose levels at specified times, and that it is important that the patient fast beforehand. The patient should also be informed that smoking, coffee, and tea are not permitted because they are stimulants and may affect the results of the test. It should be emphasized that many patients find the whole test boring and tedious, so they should be encouraged to bring a book to read, knitting, or some other occupation with them, to alleviate this. It is important that the patient feel relaxed and free from stress, as increased physical activity and mental stress may affect the results.

The nurse should explain to the patient that he may feel weak and dizzy, and may sweat during the test, but that this is usually transient.

It is important that the patient be provided with the necessary urine containers. He should also be encouraged to drink plenty of water to help him provide the urine specimens.

Once the specimens have been obtained, the nurse should ensure that each one is correctly labelled with the patient's name and the date and time it was collected.

The nurse is often the ideal person to instruct the patient how to perform finger-prick blood sampling. This increases the patient's involvement in ultimately controlling his own blood sugar requirements. This is not a painful procedure if it is carried out correctly, although initially patients may be understandably anxious about inflicting pain on themselves. There are various devices for puncturing the skin and obtaining small but sufficient amounts of blood for adequate measurement. With most reagent strips one drop of blood is all that is required. By spending time with the patient and family the nurse should be able to assist in teaching them this simple technique, but she should appreciate that nurses often have difficulty in performing these tests themselves (Hilton, 1982).

Adrenal glands

These two glands lie on top of the kidneys. They have the ability to secrete many hormones: the inner medulla of the glands secretes adrenaline and noradrenaline, and the outer cortex secretes glucocorticoids (i.e. cortisol), mineralocorticoids (i.e. aldosterone), androgens and oestrogens.

VANILLYLMANDELIC ACID (VMA) TEST

Tumours of the adrenal medulla (phaeochromocytoma) produce catecholamines (adrenaline and noradrenaline) which result in high blood pressure. The metabolites of these circulating catecholamines are excreted in the urine. The major metabolite of these catecholamines is VMA, and it is the one most conveniently measured.

Certain drugs interfere with the estimation of VMA, including barbiturates, salicylates, sulphonamides, and anti-hypertensive agents such as methyldopa. Certain foods also exert an influence, including tea, coffee, bananas, chocolate, and citrus fruit. Therefore, in order to obtain an accurate test result, the patient should be given a vanilla-free diet for at least 48 hours before the test starts. Certain drugs, or all of them, may be restricted if the physician wishes.

A 24-hour urine is collected in a specially labelled container which has in it a preservative, usually 20 ml of concentrated hydrochloric acid.

Nursing implications

It is important that the patient be given adequate advice and information about this test, particularly with regard to avoiding vanilla-containing foods and drugs. Such advice should be given in writing before the test.

The procedure for collecting the urine specimens should be carefully explained to the patient who should be shown where the urine specimen container is, and where the urinals are. He should be informed about the preservative, when the collection begins, the need to drink plenty of fluids during the 24-hour period (unless contraindicated), and the need to avoid excessive physical activity or mental stress which may affect the results by causing an increase in the secretion of adrenaline and nor-adrenaline.

The purpose of the test should be explained in simple terms: i.e., 'to help to find out what is causing the high blood pressure'. The explanation should include information about the actual collection of urine. The 24-hour collection begins after the patient urinates. The first sample is discarded, but all subsequent specimens are collected until 24 hours have passed. If one is accidentally discarded, the laboratory should be informed to see whether the collection should be started again.

Once the 24-hour collection is complete, the nurse should ensure that the container is correctly labelled with the patient's name and the date and time the collection was started and finished.

After completion, the patient is permitted to have the foods and drugs which were restricted during the preparation of the test.

There is a whole range of investigations pertinent to the endocrine system. Many of them are based on a small blood sample, but some are much more sophisticated. However, they are not all mentioned here because the amount of nursing involved is minimal.

References and further reading

Harris, G. (1983) The endocrine system. *Nursing* 2, 13, 359–362.
Hilton, B. A. (1982) Nurses' performance and interpretation of urine testing and capillary blood glucose monitoring measures, *J. Adv. Nurs.* 7, 509–521.
Kelly, B. A. (1979) Nurses' knowledge of glycosuria testing in diabetes mellitus. *Nurs. Res.* 28, 316–319.

7
Investigations Associated with the Urinary Tract

URINARY TRACT

The urinary tract consists of the two kidneys and their ureters, the bladder and the urethra. The functions of the urinary tract are to maintain homeostasis and to produce and excrete urine.

The main problems that occur in the urinary tract which result in the patient requiring investigation are due to obstruction or infection. Such problems include pain, colic, and disturbances of micturition.

Investigations associated with the urinary tract are often perceived as embarrassing and distressing by the patient, so the nurse has to use her skills to the full to allay such feelings.

Kidneys

The kidneys are located on either side of the vertebral column and receive their blood supply from the renal arteries, which originate from the abdominal aorta. Blood is drained by the renal veins, which lead into the inferior vena cava. Each kidney consists of about one million functional units called nephrons, which form the urine by filtering waste products, along with excess water and electrolytes. The prime function of the kidneys, therefore, is the excretion of metabolites and the regulation of water and electrolytes.

INTRAVENOUS PYELOGRAPHY (IVP)

This investigation permits the kidneys, ureters, and bladder to be outlined by injecting a radio opaque dye. The dye is filtered out by the glomeruli, and then passed through the renal tubules, the whole process being viewed by fluoroscopy. X-rays are taken at regular intervals.

Intravenous pyelograms are performed for the location of obstructions such as stones, tumours, and cysts; assessment of the effects of trauma to the urinary tract; and the diagnosis of kidney diseases such as polycystic kidney, congenital absence or malposition of the kidney.

Intravenous pyelograms are performed in the X-ray department by a radiologist. The procedure takes about 30–45 minutes.

The procedure and its purpose are explained to the patient, who is then asked to sign a consent form. It is important that the bowel is clear so that good visualization of the upper urinary tract can be achieved. An aperient is usually given the night before, and an enema on the day of the investigation. The patient is not usually fasted as a rule, but fluid may be restricted so that good quality X-rays of the dye can be obtained.

The patient is asked to remove any dentures, jewellery, and clothing, and to wear a gown. The nurse escorts him to the department and helps him onto the hard X-ray table, where he is asked to lie in the supine position. The radiologist injects the dye into a peripheral vein and X-ray films are taken at specific times, once the passage of the dye through the upper urinary tract is shown under fluoroscopy.

Nursing implications

The main problem with this investigation is the discomfort the patient experiences from the injection of dye. Nowadays, the injection is usually given slowly (over 2 minutes) to avoid the unpleasant flush or burning sensation, nausea, and headache that often accompany fast injections. The patient should be informed that such sensations may occur, but reassured that they are only transient. The patient should also be given information about the equipment, staff, department where the procedure takes place, and probable outcome. The purpose should be explained in simple terms: i.e., 'to see if the kidneys are normal' or 'to observe the size, shape, and structure of the urinary tract'.

The patient should be informed that he will be lying on a hard table and X-ray films will be taken at intervals, often in the dark. If any fluid restrictions are thought necessary, the patient should be told exactly what he can have and what he should avoid. He should be encouraged to ask questions or express any worries, and asked if he wishes to empty his bladder before the test and afterwards, as he may be too embarrassed to ask in case it interferes with the procedure.

Once the procedure is completed, the patient should be escorted back to the ward and encouraged to drink fluids. The injection site should be inspected to make sure there is no bleeding or haematoma.

RETROGRADE PYELOGRAPHY

This investigation permits radiological viewing of the kidneys, ureters, and bladder by the injection of a small amount of radio-opaque dye through a catheter into the ureters and renal pelvis.

Retrograde pyelograms are performed after, or in place of, intravenous pyelograms. Viewing with this technique is better because the dye is injected directly. It is also used for demonstrating any anatomical structure in the urinary tract.

Retrograde pyelograms are performed in the operating theatre by a urologist. The procedure takes about 45–60 minutes.

The procedure and its purpose are explained to the patient, who is then asked to sign a consent form. The investigation may be performed under a local anaesthetic or a general anaesthetic; whichever is chosen by the urologist, the nurse should inform the patient well beforehand. The patient is usually fasted 6–8 hours before the investigation. If a local anaesthetic is used, a sedative or narcotic analgesic may be prescribed and given beforehand, in order to make the patient feel more relaxed and less anxious.

The patient is asked to remove any dentures, jewellery, and clothing, and to wear a gown. The nurse escorts him to the operating theatre, where he is helped onto the hard table and is usually placed in the lithotomy position (feet and legs in stirrups). The urologist inserts a ureteral catheter into the renal pelvis, a dye is injected under fluoroscopy, and X-ray films are taken.

Nursing implications

The nursing care and preparation of the patient for a retrograde pyelogram will be centred on the choice of anaesthetic that is given to the patient. The patient should be informed at the start what type of anaesthetic will be given, as well as about fasting, preparation, procedure, and outcome. Information about the department where the investigation takes place, its duration, the staff and equipment involved, sensations to be expected, and anticipated findings are important in order to reduce the patient's anxiety and fear and increase his cooperation. The purpose should be explained in simple terms: i.e., 'to see if there are any stones in the urinary tract', or 'to find the cause of the kidney problem'.

The patient should be informed that he will be lying on a hard table with his feet and legs in stirrups and that a catheter will be inserted into the ureter and a dye injected, followed by X-ray filming. He should be encouraged to ask questions or express any worries or fears. He should be asked if he wishes to empty his bladder before the test. If the test is being done under a local anaesthetic, he should be told that he is likely to feel pressure with the insertion of the cystoscope (which is required for inserting the ureteral catheter), and may feel the urge to pass urine. However, there should be no pain, only a little discomfort.

Once the procedure is completed, the patient should be encouraged to rest, and offered analgesia for any pain or discomfort. The patient should not stand up or walk immediately after his legs have been removed from the stirrups as he may feel dizzy or faint.

The nurse should carefully monitor the patient's urine output, record the volume, and observe for haematuria. A small amount of blood in the urine is common. She should encourage an increased intake of fluids in order to reduce any burning on micturition. Any signs or symptoms of infection should be reported to the doctor. Sometimes prophylactic antibiotics are prescribed to reduce the likelihood of infection. However, the patient should be informed that a slight burning sensation when voiding is considered normal for the first day or two.

RENAL BIOPSY

In this investigation a specially designed needle is inserted through the skin and into the kidney to obtain a tissue sample, which is examined in the histology laboratory.

Renal biopsy is performed for diagnosing the cause of

glomerulonephritis, diagnosing malignancy, and evaluating the amount of rejection that occurs after renal transplantation.

This investigation is performed in a clinic, or more commonly on the ward, by a physician. The procedure takes about 15 minutes.

The kidney is highly vascular, so, prior to the biopsy the patient's blood is analysed for bleeding, clotting, prothrombin times, and platelet counts. The blood is then grouped and cross-matched in case haemorrhage occurs.

An intravenous pyelogram is usually performed before the biopsy to ascertain the position and anatomy of the kidney. The patient is fasted for 6 hours before the procedure. Fluoroscopy is often used for accurately guiding the biopsy needle.

The procedure and its purpose are explained to the patient. It is important to make him fully aware of the procedure and its potential dangers. He is then asked to sign a consent form. He should be asked if he wishes to pass urine before the procedure. If he is very anxious, a sedative may be required. The patient is then asked to lie in the prone position with a sandbag or pillow under the abdomen to straighten the spine. Under aseptic conditions, the skin overlying the kidney is infiltrated with a local anaesthetic. The patient is asked to hold his breath and the physician inserts the biopsy needle into the kidney and obtains the specimen. The needle is removed and pressure is applied to the puncture site for about 15 minutes. A sterile dressing is applied and the patient is placed on his back and encouraged to rest.

Nursing implications

Many patients are anxious about this investigation. However, such an understandable reaction can be allayed if the patient is given a careful explanation about the procedure, sensations to be expected, equipment used, and probable outcome. The patient should be informed that some discomfort is involved, but that the procedure is not painful, largely because of the local anaesthetic. However, the discomfort will be worse when the biopsy needle is inserted.

The purpose of the investigation should be explained in simple terms: i.e., 'to examine a piece of kidney tissue to see if it is normal'. The patient should be told to keep still during the procedure and to hold his breath when the doctor inserts the needle. It is important to reassure the patient by stressing that the procedure is safe, and by being optimistic but realistic about the outcome.

Once the procedure is completed, the nurse should apply a sterile dressing to the puncture site and explain to the patient the need to lie on his back, both to apply pressure and to rest. The nurse should ensure that the patient feels comfortable, and encourage him to drink large amounts of fluid. She should ensure that he empties his bladder and inspect all urine for haematuria. Although the urine will contain small amounts of blood initially, this will usually cease after the first 12–24 hours.

The main complication of this investigation is haemorrhage, and the nurse should observe the puncture site for bleeding. Regular recordings of the pulse and blood pressure are essential.

The patient should be instructed to avoid any strenuous activities, such as heavy lifting, contact sports, or other activities which may cause sudden movement of the kidney, for at least 2 weeks.

CYSTOSCOPY

This is an investigation which permits direct viewing of the urethra and bladder by inserting a hollow, lighted, telescopic tube (cystoscope) through the urethra into the bladder. Biopsy forceps, scissors, or a cytology brush can also be inserted through the instrument.

Cystoscopy is performed to diagnose, inspect, or obtain biopsy specimens (i.e. small renal calculi) of the ureter, bladder, or urethra. It is also performed to measure bladder capacity and to dilate the urethra and ureters.

Cystoscopy is performed in the operating theatre or cystoscopy clinic by a urologist. The procedure takes about 25 minutes.

The procedure and its purpose are explained to the patient, who is then asked to sign a consent form. The investigation may be performed under a local anaesthetic or a general anaesthetic; if the latter, the patient must obviously fast, and any fluids are given intravenously. If a local anaesthetic is used, a sedative or narcotic analgesic may be prescribed and given beforehand, in order to make the patient more relaxed and less anxious.

The patient is asked to remove any dentures, jewellery, and clothing, and to wear a gown. The nurse escorts him to the operating theatre, and helps him onto the operating table. He is usually placed in the lithotomy position (feet and legs in stirrups); the cystoscope is then introduced.

Nursing implications

The patient should be informed what type of anaesthetic will be used, and be advised about fasting and premedication. He should also be given information about the department where the investigation will take place, its duration, the staff and equipment involved, sensations to be expected, and probable outcome. The purpose should be explained in simple terms: i.e., 'to look at the interior of the bladder to see if it is normal'. He should be given the opportunity to ask questions or express any concern or worries. Women in particular may find this procedure distressing and highly personal, and the nurse should be sensitive to her feelings.

The patient should be informed that he will be lying on a hard operating table with his feet and legs in stirrups, and that a hollow, telescopic tube will be inserted into the urethra and along to the bladder to examine it. He should be asked if he wishes to pass urine before the test. If the test is being done under a local anaesthetic he should be told that he will feel pressure with the insertion of the cystoscope and possibly the urge to pass urine, but that there will be no pain, only a little discomfort.

Once the procedure is completed, the patient will probably want to rest, and should be encouraged to do so. Any pain or discomfort should be relieved with analgesia. The patient should avoid standing up suddenly or walking after he has left the table as he may feel faint or dizzy.

The nurse should carefully monitor the patient's urine output and record any haematuria. Although a small amount of blood in the urine is common, frank haematuria should be reported. She should also encourage increased fluid intake to reduce any burning sensations on micturition, and carefully observe the urine output. Any signs or symptoms of infection should be reported to the doctor. Antibiotic cover may have been prescribed to reduce the possibility of infection. However, the patient should be informed that a slight burning sensation when voiding is considered normal for the first day or two.

CYSTOGRAPHY

This investigation permits imaging of the bladder by instilling a radio-opaque dye through a urinary catheter under fluoroscopy. The filling and emptying of the bladder is recorded on video.

Cystograms are performed to detect filling defects of the bladder which may indicate tumours, fistulas, rupture, or a neurogenic bladder. They are carried out in the X-ray department, or special clinic, by a radiologist or urologist. The procedure takes from 15–30 minutes.

The procedure and its purpose are explained to the patient, who is asked to wear a hospital gown and comfortable footwear. Any jewellery should be removed for safe keeping. The nurse then escorts the patient to the department. Unless one is already in place, a catheter is inserted into the bladder via the urethra. Dye is then introduced into the bladder through the catheter, and X-ray films are taken. The catheter is usually removed while the bladder is full and filming takes place during micturition (micturating cystogram). This enables the radiologist or urologist to detect any poor bladder muscle tone and whether there is any reflux up the ureters (vesico-ureteric reflux) while the bladder is emptying.

Nursing implications

This is an embarrassing and generally unpleasant experience for the patient. The nurse must therefore use her social skills to the full in informing and reassuring the patient about the procedure. He should be told that a urinary catheter will be inserted and a dye introduced through it into the bladder, and that he will be expected to pass urine whilst being filmed, and in the presence of others (members of staff). It should be stressed that this is a relatively common investigation and that the staff are used to the reactions of the patient and fully appreciate his embarrassment. The patient should also be told about the duration of the test, the likely sensations he will experience, and the outcome. It should be made clear that although the procedure is not painful, the catheterization may cause some discomfort. The purpose of the investigation should also be explained in simple terms: i.e., 'to look at the bladder while it is filling and emptying'.

The patient should be informed that he may have to wait quite a while in the department, so it would be advisable to take a book to read. The nurse should ensure that the patient's dignity is preserved at all times and that he feels able to ask questions or express concern or worries. The patient should be allowed to watch the X-ray screen to see what is happening. Many patients express great interest in their own investigations; this should not be discouraged, and any questions should be answered truthfully.

Once the procedure is completed, the patient should be warned that his urine may be bloodstained. The nurse should carefully observe and record the patient's urine output and haematuria, and should encourage an increased fluid intake to reduce the chance of infection and to flush out any remaining dye. Any signs or symptoms of infection should be noted. The risk of subsequent infection from this investigation can be high and prophylactic antibiotics are often prescribed to reduce this.

RENAL ARTERIOGRAPHY (RENAL ANGIOGRAPHY)

This investigation permits imaging of the renal arteries by introduction of a catheter and a radio-opaque dye with the aid of fluoroscopy.

Renal arteriograms are performed for the diagnosis of renal stenosis and, to a lesser extent, tumours, cysts, and aneurysms. They are carried out in the X-ray department or operating theatre, by a radiologist or urologist. The procedure takes from 1 to 2 hours.

The procedure and its purpose are explained to the patient, who is asked to sign a consent form. The catheter insertion site (usually the femoral) is shaved and the patient is encouraged to have a bath. He is also asked to fast for 6 hours beforehand. Premedication—i.e. sedative or narcotic analgesic—is prescribed and given.

The patient is asked to remove any dentures, jewellery, and clothing, and to wear a gown. He is escorted to the department and helped onto the hard X-ray table, and asked to lie in the supine position. The catheter insertion site is aseptically prepared and a local anaesthetic is given. The radiologist or urologist performs a femoral arterial stab, the catheter is inserted, and the dye is injected rapidly. Serial X-ray films are then taken to show the origins of the renal arteries and any accessory arteries.

Nursing implications

Anxiety about the thought of a catheter being inserted and a dye injected into the renal arteries can be allayed by careful explanation about the procedure, equipment, sensations to be expected, staff involved, and the department where the procedure will take place. The purpose should be explained in simple terms: i.e., 'to look at the blood vessels in the kidneys'. The patient should be encouraged to express any concern or fear.

The nurse needs to explain to the patient the sensations he is likely to experience: i.e., a warm, flushing sensation when the dye is injected. The patient should be given an account of the intended procedure in sequence: i.e., a doctor will inject a dye into an artery in the groin; the area will be numbed, and a catheter will be inserted. He should be told that the procedure is not painful, apart from the arterial puncture, but that discomfort may occur at times. He should also be told that he will have to lie still on a hard table, and that films will be taken at intervals in the dark, but he will be able to talk and watch the filming.

Once the procedure is completed, pressure must be applied at the insertion site for about 15 minutes. The site should be observed for swelling or haematoma. A small dressing is usually applied. Attention should be paid to any strange sensations such as numbness, tingling, or pain. The patient should rest in bed for about 12 hours and should not move his legs very much as this may result in haemorrhage or swelling. The patient's blood pressure and pulse rate should be recorded at 15-minute intervals.

References and further reading

Cameron, J. S., Russell, A. M. E. & Sale, D. N. T. (1979) *Nephrology for Nurses*. London: Heinemann.

Goodinson, S. M. (1984) Renal function: an overview. *Nursing* 2, 29, 843–852.

Tinckler, L. (1984) The urinary system. *Nurs. Mirror* **158**, 7, 22–26.

Wallis, C. M. (1984) The collection and testing of urine. *Nursing* 2, 29, 853–854.

8
Investigations Associated with the Female Reproductive System

REPRODUCTIVE SYSTEM

In the female the reproductive system consists of the ovaries, fallopian tubes, uterus, and vagina. The main problems that occur in the female reproductive system which result in the patient requiring investigation are due to disease and trauma. Such problems include pain, disturbances of bleeding, and abnormal discharges.

Investigations associated with the female reproductive system are often perceived as very stressful by the patient. Such stress and fear is understandable. Many gynaecological problems are associated with fear of loss or damage to the function of the reproductive organs, worry about sexuality and the effects on intimate relationships, and concern about pregnancy. Paramount is the fear of cancer, as many patients who attend for investigation know that this is a possible diagnosis. Therefore, the care and the support these patients require when undergoing investigation demands a high level of nursing skill. Some patients will wish to discuss their fears and anxieties, others will not. The nurse should be able to recognize this. Her main skill will be that of a good and attentive listener. If she cannot answer some of the patient's specific questions she should refer her to the appropriate expert.

Sensitivity, empathy, confidentiality, privacy, and comfort are all important in the care of these patients.

Reproductive organs

The vagina is a muscular canal which leads from the introitus to a hollow, muscular, pear-shaped organ, the uterus. This lies almost at right angles to the vagina. The lower end of the uterus, the cervix, projects into the vagina for nearly half its length. Two thin muscular tubes (fallopian tubes) link the uterus to the peritoneal cavity. Here, on the back of the broad ligament, lie the ovaries, which are the female sex glands. These secrete the hormones oestrogen and progesterone and, in the adult, provide germ cells.

CERVICAL SMEAR

In this investigation the cervix is exposed by the insertion of a vaginal speculum and cervical epithelial cells are obtained by scraping the cervix with a spatula.

Cervical smears are performed for detecting the presence of cervical cancer. They are said to be 95% accurate. It has been suggested that a cervical smear should be carried out routinely on all women over the age of 18 at annual intervals.

Cervical smears are performed in the family planning clinic, general practice surgery, or on a ward in a private examination room, by a doctor or experienced nurse. The procedure takes about 5–10 minutes.

The procedure and its purpose are explained to the patient, who is asked to undress from the waist downwards. She is then asked to lie on the examining table, or couch, with her legs drawn up and knees apart. The doctor (or nurse) palpates the abdomen, inspects the external genitalia, and then carefully introduces a warmed and lubricated speculum into the vagina to inspect the cervix. Swabs and smears may then be obtained.

Nursing implications

Although this is a common investigation it is, nevertheless, a traumatic experience for many women. Patient cooperation is essential and this can be encouraged by careful explanation, reassurance, and support.

If the examination is to be performed by a male doctor, a female nurse must be present as a chaperone. Her prime responsibility is to the patient. She should assure the patient that this is an examination and not a form of treatment, and that it is painless, quick, and will be carried out in privacy. The purpose should be explained in simple terms: i.e., 'to see if there are any abnormal cells in the cervix'. However, the actual procedure should be explained in sequence in some detail, as this will help to reduce the patient's anxiety.

The nurse should find out whether the patient has undergone this investigation before and whether she is menstruating. If she is, the examination may be postponed. She should be asked to pass urine before the test.

The examination should be conducted in privacy, preferably in a private room. The patient is asked to undress from the waist downwards and is helped onto the examining couch. If a gynaecological examination couch is used, the patient's feet rest in stirrups. Whatever position is used, the nurse should ensure that dignity is maintained by ensuring the patient is warm, comfortable, and well covered by a blanket to minimize exposure. The nurse can allay fears by careful listening and sensible conversation. Touch is very important, and many women prefer to hold or grip a nurse's hand or arm.

Once the procedure is completed, the patient should be offered tissues to wipe herself dry. She should be helped to dress and told when the results of the test will be available and how she can obtain them. This is very important.

The cells obtained by the smear are transferred onto a microscopic slide and fixed, correctly labelled, and sent to the laboratory for analysis.

COLPOSCOPY

This investigation permits direct viewing of the vagina and cervix using a microscope with a light source and a magnifying lens (colposcope).

Colposcopy is performed for identifying vaginal and cervical lesions which would be missed by the naked eye. It is carried out in a gynaecology clinic by a gynaecologist. The procedure takes from 5 to 15 minutes.

The procedure and purpose are explained to the patient, who is asked to undress, wear a gown and lie on the examination couch in the lithotomy position. A warm lubricated speculum is introduced into the vagina to inspect the vagina and cervix. Secretions and debris are removed with a swab, and acetic acid (usually 3% solution) is applied to the vaginal and cervical epithelium. This accentuates the difference between normal and abnormal tissue. Photographs are often taken and, if there is a suspicion of abnormal tissue, a biopsy may be taken. Pressure at the biopsy site or cautery may be used to stop the bleeding.

Nursing implications

Most women are very anxious at the prospect of undergoing this investigation. Careful explanation, encouragement, and support are needed to achieve the patient's cooperation, which is essential if the investigation is to be successful.

The nurse should point out that colposcopy is purely a diagnostic procedure and not a form of treatment. She should explain the purpose in simple terms: i.e., 'to look at the vagina and cervix in more detail', or 'to see if there are any possible tissue changes in the cervix'. The procedure should be explained in detail and in sequence. It should be stressed that the investigation will take place in privacy, that it will be relatively quick (i.e. not more than 15 minutes), painless (unless a biopsy is taken, in which case some discomfort may occur), and that only the members of staff necessary will be present. The explanation should include information about the lithotomy position (i.e. feet supported in stirrups), the instruments used (speculum and colposcope), and the fact that the colposcope is not inserted into the vagina but is used to focus and magnify cervical tissue. She should also be warned that photographs and a biopsy may be taken.

The nurse should ensure that the patient is safe, comfortable, warm, and not exposed unnecessarily. She should listen attentively to expressions of the patient's worries or concern and offer advice or refer the problem to an expert. Touch should also be used as a therapeutic measure as this plays a big part in comforting and reassuring the patient.

Once the procedure is completed, the patient should be provided with tampons or a sanitary towel because of the bleeding that may occur if a biopsy has been performed. She should be informed that she may have bleeding for a short while, but if it is heavy she should get in touch with the gynaecologist. She should be advised that it is wise not to have intercourse for a few days (i.e. 5–7 days), until the biopsy site has healed. She should also be told when the results of the test will be available and how she can obtain them.

LAPAROSCOPY

This investigation permits direct viewing of the abdominal and pelvic cavities, using a fibreoptic instrument with light source (laparoscope) inserted through the abdominal wall and into the peritoneum.

Laparoscopy is performed for the diagnosis of pelvic adhesions, ovarian cysts and tumours, and other causes of infertility. Procedures such as organ biopsy and tubal ligation can be easily performed with the laparoscope.

Laparoscopy is performed in the operating theatre by a gynaecologist. The procedure takes from 15 to 30 minutes.

The patient's blood is sampled for haemoglobin, grouping, and cross-matching, in case a transfusion is required for surgery. A clear bowel is needed and this is achieved by aperients or an enema given the night before. The abdomen is shaved to remove hair from around the umbilicus and upper pubic region, and a bath is encouraged on the morning of the procedure.

The procedure and its purpose are explained to the patient, who is asked to sign a consent form. The investigation is performed under a general anaesthetic and the patient should be informed of this and fasted for 6 hours beforehand. The patient should be asked if she wishes to pass urine. She should then be asked to remove any dentures, jewellery, and clothing, and to wear a gown. Premedication is given about 1 hour before the procedure. This will promote relaxation and reduce secretions.

The nurse escorts the patient to the operating theatre where she is transferred onto the hard table and is placed in the Trendelenburg (head-down) or modified lithotomy position, after the anaesthetic has been administered. The purpose of the positioning is to ensure that the abdominal contents move away from the pelvic contents, thus permitting better viewing of the pelvic organs. The skin is aseptically cleaned and a small incision is made below the umbilicus for the insertion of the laparoscope. Between 3 and 4 litres of gas (usually carbon dioxide) are introduced into the abdominal cavity to distend it and facilitate viewing. After this, a trocar within a cannula is introduced. The trocar is removed and the laparoscope is introduced and the pelvic and abdominal structures are examined. When inspection (or a procedure such as tubal ligation) is completed, the laparoscope is removed and the gas released. The incision site is closed with a suture and covered with a small sterile dressing.

Nursing implications

Most women are anxious and sometimes frightened about undergoing this procedure. Careful explanation will allay such fears, relax the patient, and gain her cooperation and trust. She should be informed that the procedure will be performed under a general anaesthetic and that she is unlikely to have any severe pain afterwards, but may have mild pain from the incision site. She should also be informed that although primarily a diagnostic procedure, surgery in the form of tubal ligation or biopsy may be carried out if the gynaecologist considers it necessary. It is important that the patient is made fully aware of this before she is asked to give her written consent.

The purpose of the investigation should be explained to the patient in simple terms: i.e., 'to look at organs in the pelvis and abdomen to see if they are normal'. She should also be informed about the actual procedure, staff and equipment involved, the place where it takes place, the duration, and the expected outcome. It is important to explain that she will need to fast beforehand and that afterwards she may feel drowsy, nauseous, and in some pain which may be persistent, and, in some cases, severe. The effects of the premedication should also be explained. The nurse should encourage the patient to express her fears and worries, and to ask questions. Those the nurse cannot answer she should refer to the appropriate expert.

Once the procedure is completed, the nurse should carry out all routine post-operative nursing measures, including maintenance of clear airway, observations of pulse rate and blood pressure, and relief of anxiety, nausea, and pain. Although there are no restrictions on food and fluid intake, it is important to ensure that the patient's gag reflex has returned before offering food or drink. Any pain should be treated immediately with analgesia. A vulval toilet may be required, and careful monitoring of urine output is important. Sometimes a dye is injected during laparoscopy to test the fallopian tubes for patency. If this has been done, the patient should be warned that the urine may be a blue/green colour, which may also appear in the vagina. A sanitary towel will prevent staining of clothes.

The nurse should be aware of possible complications such as haemorrhage and perforation, and carefully observe pulse rate and blood pressure. The puncture site should be observed for bleeding or haematoma. The sutures are removed as soon as the wound has healed.

Many women are anxious about the outcome of this procedure.

The results should be given to the patient as soon as possible. If they are not immediately available, the patient should be informed how and when she can obtain them. She may also be worried about resuming sexual intercourse, and returning to work. If a biopsy has been taken she should be advised to avoid intercourse for about 5–7 days, by which time the site will have healed. However, in general, most women can be advised to resume sexual relationships, and work, when they feel comfortable and able to do so.

AMNIOCENTESIS

In this investigation a needle is inserted through the abdominal and uterine walls into the amniotic cavity to withdraw fluid for laboratory analysis.

Amniocentesis is performed for assessing the sex and maturity of the fetus, genetic and chromosomal abnormalities such as Down's syndrome, or anatomical abnormalities. It is performed during the 14th–16th weeks of pregnancy.

Amniocentesis is performed in an obstetric clinic by an obstetrician. The procedure takes from 20 to 30 minutes.

The procedure and its purpose are explained to the patient, who is asked to sign a consent form. The investigation is performed on an out-patient basis under aseptic conditions. The patient is asked to undress, wear a gown, and to pass urine before the procedure to prevent the bladder being punctured. The patient is then asked to lie on the examining couch in the supine position. The fetal heart is auscultated and the placenta is located by ultrasound so that the site for the needle insertion can be chosen. The skin site is then aseptically cleansed and infiltrated with local anaesthetic. A needle with stilette is inserted, often with ultrasound guidance. The stilette is removed and a small sterile syringe is attached. From 5 to 15 ml of amniotic fluid is withdrawn, and the needle is then removed. A small dressing is applied to the puncture site; the amniotic fluid is placed in a container, correctly labelled, and sent to the laboratory for analysis.

Nursing implications

Many women are extremely anxious about undergoing this

investigation, but it is the outcome of the test rather than the actual procedure which concerns them. Their concern is obvious, and the nurse should be sensitive to it. She should recognize the reasons why amniocentesis is indicated and encourage the patient to express concern or ask questions.

The procedure should be explained in detail to both the patient and her partner, and it should be emphasized that amniocentesis is not a routine screening test. The nurse should tell them that great care is taken to minimize the risk to her and the fetus; that the procedure is quickly carried out, is safe and painless, apart from the injection of local anaesthetic. The safety of ultrasound (Stark et al., 1984) should also be stressed. The purpose should be explained in simple terms: i.e., 'to detect possible birth defects'. Although risks are rare, it is important that the doctor warns her of potential problems, such as infection or bleeding.

It is important that the nurse should be a good listener, and supportive, and able to recognize the concerns of the patient and her partner and empathize with them. Because they will be worried about the results of the test, they should be told how and when to obtain them. It is relevant to find out the patient's views on abortion before amniocentesis is even suggested.

Breast

The breasts (mammary glands) consist of glandular and fatty tissue, and are situated on the anterior wall of the thorax. The development and function of these glands are influenced by a wide variety of endocrine factors, the most important being prolactin and oestrogens.

The breasts play an important role in the concept of femininity and in a woman's body image. Any damage to them will usually result in severe psychological problems.

MAMMOGRAPHY

This X-ray investigation permits the detection of cysts or tumours in the breast. It is performed when clinical examination or thermography reveals a suspicious lump. A low-energy X-ray beam is used to reduce the amount of radiation received by the patient.

Mammography is performed in the X-ray department or breast screening clinic by a radiographer. The procedure takes about 20 minutes.

The procedure and its purpose are explained to the patient. It is contraindicated during pregnancy, so this should be checked with the patient. No special preparation is necessary. The patient is asked to undress from the neck to the waist. She is also asked to remove any necklaces and to wear a gown which is open at the front. She is asked to identify the lump in the breast if one is present. The patient usually stands up (but sometimes is seated), resting the breast on an X-ray plate, against which the breast is compressed. The patient is then asked to hold her breath and a number of films are taken from different views.

Nursing implications

Although this is a routine investigation, many women are under-standably concerned and worried about it, particularly with regard to outcome. The purpose should be explained in simple terms: i.e., 'to see what the palpable lump is', or 'a routine breast examination'. The nurse should be a good listener and suppor-tive. She should assure the patient that this is a common investigation which is quickly performed, that it is safe and causes no pain, only a little discomfort when the breast is compressed. However, in some patients such pressure may be unexpectedly painful. She should be told not to worry or be alarmed if additional films are required.

Because they will be worried about the outcome of the test, the patient and partner should be told how and when to obtain the results. These are usually available within a few days.

It is a good idea to instruct and encourage the patient to undertake self-examination of the breast for lumps.

References and further reading

Ray, C., Grover, J. & Wisniewski, T. (1984) Nurses' perceptions of early breast cancer and mastectomy, and their psychological implications, and of the role of health professionals in providing support. *Int. J. Nurs. Stud.* **21**, 101–111.

Shorthouse, M. & Brush, M. (1981) *Gynaecology in Nursing Practice*. London: Baillière Tindall.

Stark, C. R., Orleans, M., Haverkamp, A. D. & Murphy, J. (1984) Short- and long-term risks after exposure to diagnostic ultrasound in utero. *Obstet. Gynecol.* **63**, 2, 194–200.

Tindall, V. (1984) Cervical cancer 1: pathology and research. *Nurs. Mirror.* **159**, 12, 16–18.

Yule, R. (1984) Cervical cancer 2: screening for prevention. *Nurs. Mirror.* **159**, 13, 37–39.

9
Investigations Associated with the Nervous System

NERVOUS SYSTEM

The nervous system, together with the endocrine system, provides most of the control functions for the body. It is unique in the vast complexity of actions that it can perform. It receives information from a wide range of sensory organs and integrates them in order to determine what responses the body will make.

The nervous system may conveniently be divided into three areas: the control centre, i.e., the brain and spinal cord (central nervous system); the nerves that extend away from the control centre, i.e., the cranial and spinal nerves (peripheral nervous system); and the nerves that regulate functions of internal organs and other body structures that cannot be controlled consciously, i.e., the sympathetic and parasympathetic nervous system (autonomic nervous system).

Investigations associated with the nervous system are often perceived by the patient as very serious and stressful. This is understandable, as many of their problems are related to changes in, or loss of, function and/or sensation. Such changes, which may be gradual or rapid in onset, are understandably frightening to the patient who is unsure whether they will be temporary or permanent. The nurse should appreciate this, and be a skilled and attentive listener. She should assess the patient's level of awareness, orientation, memory and mood, which may be disturbed.

LUMBAR PUNCTURE AND EXAMINATION OF THE CEREBROSPINAL FLUID

This investigation involves the insertion of a needle into the subarachnoid space of the spinal column, in order to measure the pressure of the space and to obtain cerebrospinal fluid (CSF) for examination in the laboratory.

The main indication for lumbar puncture and CSF examination is to confirm the diagnosis of subarachnoid haemorrhage, meningitis, or cerebral or spinal-cord tumours. It may also be performed for the introduction of drugs or anaesthetics. It is not indicated if the CSF pressure is thought to be raised (thus, it may be contraindicated in cerebral tumour). This investigation is performed under a local anaesthetic on the ward by a physician. The procedure takes about 10 minutes.

The procedure and its purpose are explained to the patient, who is asked to sign a consent form. The patient is asked to undress and wear a gown, and a bath is usually encouraged. No fasting or sedation is normally required. The patient empties the bladder beforehand and is then carefully positioned on the bed. He is asked to lie on his side with his back near the edge of the bed. It is important that the lumbar spine is flexed as fully as possible to maximize the space between the vertebrae. This is achieved by asking the patient to draw his knees up towards his abdomen, and to flex the head and trunk.

The skin surface is aseptically prepared and infiltrated with local anaesthetic. The physician chooses a vertebral interspace anywhere between L2 and S1 (spinal cord ends at L2). The spinal needle with stilette is carefully inserted through the skin and into the spinal canal. The stilette is removed, the sterile manometer is attached to the needle, and the pressure is recorded. Three sterile bottles are filled with CSF (5–10 ml) and sent to the laboratory immediately.

Examination of CSF in the laboratory usually includes evaluation for the presence of blood, bacteria, malignant cells, glucose, protein, and chloride.

The spinal needle is removed and pressure is placed over the puncture site.

Nursing implications

Most patients are anxious and frightened that this may be a painful procedure which may result in permanent damage. They are often particularly frightened that the spinal needle may cause paralysis. It is important that such fears are allayed by careful and sensitive explanation, which will cover factors such as the actual procedure, equipment, sensations to be expected, duration, staff involved, and probable outcome. The patient should be made to understand that some degree of discomfort is often involved with the actual insertion of the spinal needle, but that the local anaesthetic will minimize this. It should be explained that the patient can assist by remaining as still as possible throughout the procedure, and that he should ask the nurse for anything he needs.

The purpose of the investigation should be explained in simple terms to the patient and relatives: i.e., 'to obtain and examine a small amount of spinal fluid for analysis in the laboratory to see if it is normal'. They should be encouraged to ask questions. They should be informed of the need for careful positioning and the reason for it. The effect and duration of the local anaesthetic should also be explained, as well as the sensations experienced when the spinal needle is inserted (usually a feeling of pressure being exerted locally), and the local anaesthetic is being injected (usually a stinging feeling).

It is also important that the patient feel safe and relatively relaxed. Care and support in maintaining the patient's position is essential. The nurse should encourage the patient in conversation, thus reassuring him and informing him of the progress of the procedure. If for some reason the procedure is performed on someone with raised intracranial pressure (i.e. due to tumour), acute respiratory distress can occur due to the pons being pushed into the foramen magnum. Artificial ventilation is then necessary.

Once the procedure is completed, the nurse should apply a sterile occlusive dressing to the puncture site. Often, an aerosol dressing is used to seal the site. The patient is made warm and comfortable and is assessed for any discomfort that may require analgesia. The patient is usually nursed lying flat with one pillow for 6–12 hours.

The patient will probably want to rest, as the procedure is rather tiring. The wound site should be checked for leakage, bleeding, or haematoma. The nurse should tell the patient that he may eat or drink normally, and that although a small amount of CSF has been removed, the body will replace this within a few days. She should also explain that headaches are common after this procedure and usually respond to rest and simple analgesia; severe symptoms accompanied by respiratory distress should be reported immediately to the physician.

The patient will be anxious about the outcome of the procedure and should be informed how and when to obtain the test results.

CEREBRAL ANGIOGRAPHY

This investigation permits imaging of the cerebral vascular system by introducing a catheter and a radio-opaque dye with the aid of fluoroscopy.

Cerebral angiograms are performed for the detection of abnormalities of the cerebral circulation such as aneurysms, occlusion, thrombosis, haematomas, or tumours. They are also performed to determine cerebral blood flow.

Cerebral angiograms are carried out in the X-ray department by a radiologist. The procedure takes from 1 to 2 hours.

The procedure and its purpose are explained to the patient, who is asked to sign a consent form. The catheter insertion site (either the femoral, brachial, or carotid) is shaved and the patient is encouraged to have a bath before the procedure. He is also asked to fast for 6 hours beforehand. Premedication—i.e. sedative or narcotic analgesic—is prescribed and given. If the patient is confused or extremely restless, a general anaesthetic may be considered more appropriate.

The patient is asked to remove any dentures, jewellery, and clothing, and to wear a gown. He is escorted to the department and helped onto the hard X-ray table, and asked to lie in the supine position. The catheter insertion site is aseptically prepared and a local anaesthetic is given. The radiologist performs an arterial stab or 'cutdown', the catheter is inserted under fluoroscopy, and the dye is injected rapidly. Serial X-ray films are then taken. The patient may be filmed in different positions: i.e. lateral and supine.

Nursing implications

Anxiety about the thought of a catheter being inserted and a dye injected into the cerebral vascular system is common and entirely understandable. However, it can be allayed by careful explanation about the procedure, equipment, sensations to be expected, staff involved, and the department where the procedure will take place. The purpose should be explained in simple terms: i.e., 'to look at the blood vessels in the brain to see if they are normal', and the patient should be encouraged to express any concern or fear.

The nurse should explain to the patient the sensations he is likely to experience: i.e., a warm, flushing sensation when the dye is injected. In more severe cases, there is a burning sensation. However, the sensations are only transient. The patient should be given an account of the intended procedure in sequence: i.e., a doctor will inject a dye into an artery in the groin (the femoral artery is commonly used); the area will be numbed and a catheter will be inserted. He should be told the procedure is not painful, apart from the arterial puncture, but discomfort may occur at times; and that he will be lying still on a hard table. Films will be taken at intervals in the dark, but he will be able to talk and watch the filming.

Once the procedure is completed, pressure must be applied at the insertion site for about 15 minutes. The site should be observed for swelling or haematoma. A small dressing is usually applied. Attention should be paid to any strange sensations such as numbness, tingling, or pain. The patient should rest in bed for at least 12 hours, flat and as still as possible. This will help to reduce headache—a common occurrence. Any pain should be relieved by analgesia and a sedative is often prescribed. The patient should be told he may eat and drink when he wants.

The nurse should record the patient's blood pressure and pulse rate at 15-minute intervals. She should carefully assess his mental state. Other observations will include the puncture site, temperature, and loss of function.

ELECTROENCEPHALOGRAPHY

The electroencephalogram (EEG) is a graphic recording of the electrical activity of the brain as detected on the skull by electrodes. This recording is displayed on moving graph paper.

The main indication for an electroencephalogram is to confirm the diagnosis of epilepsy. It is also used to diagnose cerebral lesions such as haemorrhage, abscesses, tumours, or thrombosis, but nowadays this is relatively uncommon, particularly with the advent of CT scanning.

This investigation is performed in the EEG department by a technician. The procedure takes from 90 minutes to 2 hours.

The procedure and its purpose are explained to the patient. It should be stressed that the EEG machine records the electrical activity of the brain, but does not send out electric currents, as some patients believe.

It is important that the patient be relaxed and follow the technician's instructions during the procedure. The patient should be given the opportunity to empty his bladder beforehand. He is then asked to sit in a chair while the electrodes are applied to the skull, either by means of a special rubber cap which holds the electrode pads in place, or directly to the scalp using contact gel. When all the electrodes are in position the patient is asked to place himself comfortably in a chair or on a couch. The EEG machine is switched on and the recording begun.

During the recording certain 'activation techniques' are commonly used in an effort to enhance abnormal brain activity. These include hyperventilation and flashing lights. Occasionally, barbiturates may be given to accentuate specific 'waves'. The patient will also be asked to keep his eyes closed for a certain period of time and then to open them in order to elicit a specific response.

Once the procedure is completed, the electrodes and cap are removed and the scalp is cleaned and dried.

Nursing implications

Any fears the patient may have about this investigation may be allayed by the knowledge that it is non-invasive, not particularly unpleasant, does not cause discomfort, and does not result in complications. These points should be explained.

The purpose of the investigation should be explained in simple terms: i.e., 'to record the electrical activity of the brain'. The procedure should also be explained to the patient with regard to body position, electrode placement, and duration. The patient should be encouraged to relax and to follow the instructions given during the recording. He should be informed that the only inconvenience is to have a lot of electrodes placed on his scalp. The actual positioning and method of application should be described and he should be warned that he may wish to have his hair washed after the investigation.

If barbiturates or other drugs have been given the effects,

duration, and side-effects should be mentioned. The patient should be advised not to drive, but should be accompanied home by a friend or relative.

PNEUMOENCEPHALOGRAPHY (AIR ENCEPHALOGRAPHY)

This investigation permits imaging of the ventricles and sub-arachnoid space by injecting air or oxygen into the lumbar subarachnoid space by lumbar puncture.

The main indications for a pneumoencephalogram are to detect tumours and atrophy of the cerebrum or cerebellum, and to assess hydrocephalus. It is a helpful investigation when CT scanning is not available, but it is less sensitive and accurate, and is invasive.

This investigation is performed in the X-ray department by a radiologist. The procedure takes from 1 to 2 hours.

The procedure and its purpose are explained to the patient, who is asked to sign a consent form. He is asked to fast for at least 6 hours beforehand. Premedication—i.e. sedative or narcotic analgesic—is prescribed and given. The investigation may be performed under a local or general anaesthetic: the latter is preferred because the procedure is painful and frightening.

The patient is asked to remove any dentures, jewellery, and clothing, and to wear a gown. He is escorted to the department where the anaesthetic is given. A lumbar puncture is then performed. About 6–8 ml of cerebrospinal fluid is withdrawn and air or oxygen (5–30 ml) is gradually introduced into the subarachnoid space. The patient, who is securely strapped to the special X-ray table, is turned in different positions in order to ensure that the air circulates throughout the ventricular spaces. X-rays are then taken.

Nursing implications

This investigation is very painful and frightening for the patient. The nurse's prime aim, therefore, is to try to allay such fears and relieve any pain. Careful explanation is essential, particularly about the actual procedure and the discomfort associated with it. Other information given to the patient will include his positioning, the equipment involved, department and staff, duration of the actual procedure, and expected outcome. The choice of anaesthetic will be made by the physician, and the patient informed so that he can be adequately prepared.

The purpose should be explained in simple terms: i.e., 'to look at the structure of the brain to see if it is normal'. The patient should be encouraged to express any fear or concern. He should be assured that measures will be taken to alleviate any discomfort. He should be told he will be strapped to a hard table and filmed in different positions. If this procedure is performed under a local anaesthetic he should be warned that he may be able to feel air being inserted and rising up, causing strange sensations and noises. However, these sensations are very common and are transient, and there is no cause for alarm. The patient will also need information about the lumbar puncture.

Once the procedure is completed, pressure must be applied at the insertion site for about 15 minutes. The site should be observed for swelling or haematoma. A small dressing is usually applied. The patient should lie flat in bed for at least 12 hours afterwards. Careful observations of pulse and blood pressure as well as mental state and pupil reactions and size are important. Headache is relatively common and is relieved with simple analgesia. Attention should be paid to strange sensations such as numbness, tingling, or pain, and also to loss of function.

Once the patient's gag reflex has returned he may start to drink and, later, gradually eat a normal diet.

MYELOGRAPHY

This investigation permits viewing of the spinal canal by injecting a radio-opaque dye into the subarachnoid space, under fluoroscopy.

The main indication for a myelogram is to detect spinal lesions such as tumours and prolapsed intervertebral discs. The entire spinal canal can be examined.

This investigation is performed in the X-ray department by a radiologist. The procedure takes from 45 to 60 minutes.

The procedure and its purpose are explained to the patient, who is asked to sign a consent form. He is also asked to fast for at least 6 hours beforehand. Premedication—i.e. sedative/narcotic analgesic and atropine—is prescribed and given. This investigation is usually performed under a local anaesthetic, but sometimes a general anaesthetic is preferred.

The patient is asked to remove any dentures, jewellery, and clothing and to wear a gown. He is escorted by the nurse to the X-ray department, where the anaesthetic is given. A lumbar puncture is then performed. About 15 ml of cerebrospinal fluid is withdrawn and 15 ml of dye is injected into the subarachnoid space. The patient, who is securely strapped to the special X-ray table, is placed in the prone position with his head tilted down. X-ray films are taken. The table is then tilted so the head is upward, and the dye is aspirated and the spinal needle is removed.

Nursing implications

This investigation is quite painful and frightening for the patient. The nurse can allay his fears by carefully explaining the actual procedure, sensations to be expected, positioning of the patient, department, staff, and equipment involved, duration, and expected outcome. The purpose should be explained in simple terms: i.e., 'to look at the structure of the spinal canal to see if it is normal'. Information should be given about positioning, i.e. he will have to lie on his abdomen, strapped to a hard X-ray table, and tilted so that the dye will fill the spinal canal. The choice of anaesthetic, the effects, duration, and side-effects of the drugs used, and the need for fasting, should also be discussed with the patient beforehand. The nurse should also ensure that the patient has the opportunity to pass urine before the procedure. Because a lumbar puncture is being performed, the patient will require information about this procedure.

Once the procedure is completed, pressure must be applied at the insertion site. A small sterile occlusive dressing is then usually applied. The nurse should observe the site for swelling or haematoma. She should advise the patient to lie flat on his back in bed for at least 12 hours. Careful observations of blood pressure, pulse, and mental state are important. She should observe for signs and symptoms of meningeal irritation, such as fever, stiff neck, headache, or photophobia, and inform the physician if these occur. However, mild headaches are common in the first 24–48 hours. A high temperature is also relatively common. But if both of these are severe, the nurse should report this. Attention should also be paid to strange sensations such as numbness, tingling, or pain, as well as loss of function.

ELECTROMYOGRAPHY

The electromyogram (EMG) is a graphic recording of the electrical activity of skeletal muscles at rest and during voluntary muscle contraction. This recording is displayed on an oscilloscope (monitor) as a waveform.

The main indication for an electromyogram is to detect such muscular disorders as muscular dystrophy, myaesthenia gravis, and myotonia. It is also used to differentiate between myopathy and neuropathy.

This investigation is usually performed in the EMG department, or in a department of neurology or physical rehabilitation, by a technician. The procedure usually takes about 20 minutes.

The procedure and its purpose are explained to the patient. It should be stressed that the EMG machine records the electrical activity of the brain, but does not send out electric currents to the patient.

It is important that the patient is relaxed and follows the technician's instructions during the procedure. No special preparation is necessary, other than asking the patient if he wishes to pass urine beforehand. He is then asked to sit in a chair or lie on a couch: the position depends on the muscle(s) to be studied. A needle that acts as a recording electrode is carefully inserted into the muscle being studied. A reference electrode is placed nearby on the skin surface. The patient is asked to relax the muscle and then slowly contract it.

Nursing implications

The purpose of the investigation should be explained in simple terms: i.e., 'to record the activity of the muscle at rest and when active'. The procedure should be explained in sequence, and the patient should be assured that there is no danger of electrocution. He should be informed that a recording needle will be inserted into the muscle being studied, but that although there will be some discomfort this will only be slight and temporary. He should be instructed to relax/contract the muscle(s) when requested by the technician; the nurse may have to demonstrate how to do this.

Drugs such as muscle relaxants, anticholinergics, and cholinergics may be withheld if the physician considers it necessary, and the nurse should inform the patient once she has ascertained what drugs, if any, he is taking.

Once the procedure is completed, the nurse should observe the puncture site for haematoma or inflammation.

NERVE CONDUCTION STUDIES

Nerve conduction studies are recordings of the conduction velocities of impulses in specific nerves. An electrical impulse is initiated at a specific site (proximal) of a nerve and a recording is made of the time it takes for the impulse to reach a second site (distal) of the same nerve. The conduction velocity can then be determined. In general, the normal conduction velocity will range from approximately 50 to 60 metres per second.

The main indications for nerve conduction studies are neuropathy or trauma of a nerve, where there will be a slowing of the conduction velocity.

This investigation is usually performed in a department of neurology or physical rehabilitation, or at the bedside, by a technician or neurologist. The procedure usually takes about 15 minutes.

The procedure and its purpose are explained to the patient. A recording electrode is placed on the skin overlying a muscle innervated solely by the nerve being studied. The conduction velocity is recorded once an electrical impulse has been initiated.

Nursing implications

The purpose of the investigation should be explained simply: i.e., 'to record the activity of a nerve when stimulated'. The procedure should be explained in sequence, and the patient assured that there is no danger of electrocution. He should be told that the procedure is painless, non-invasive, and quick.

References and further reading

Duthie, J. (1983) The nervous system—structure and function. *Nursing*
    2, 15, 431–434.
Purchese, G. & Allan, D. (1984) *Neuromedical and Neurosurgical Nursing*.
    London: Baillière Tindall.
Snyder, M. Ed. (1983) *A Guide to Neurological and Neurosurgical Nursing*.
    New York: Wiley.

10
Miscellaneous Investigations

Many medical investigations cannot be conveniently grouped under the headings for previous chapters, so will be considered separately here.

RADIOGRAPHY

X-rays are a form of electromagnetic energy of a very short wave-length which have the ability to penetrate tissues. Various tissues and substances differ in their ability to resist the penetration of X-rays: air, water, fat, and bone will absorb varying degrees of radiation. Air has less density, causing dark images on the X-ray film, whilst bone has a high density, causing light images on the film.

X-ray dosages are usually measured in units called 'rads'. When X-rays are used for diagnostic purposes (as opposed to therapeutic purposes) the doses are very low and are limited to a specific area of the body.

X-rays are one of the investigations most often requested by the physician. They are painless (unless used in conjunction with contrast media, which may cause some discomfort), relatively safe (Russell, 1984), easy and quick to perform, but often frightening for the patient.

A recent study of patients' attitudes towards X-ray examinations involving contrast media (Allan and Armstrong, 1984) found that nearly half of the patients studied reported being worried about the unpleasantness and nearly two thirds about the possible findings. Most patients, especially those who were worried about the actual procedure, would have liked more information about why they were having the investigation.

Plain X-ray films are commonly performed on the chest and, to a lesser extent, the abdomen, skull, and limbs, in order to study bones, including bone disease, fractures, maturity, and size. Contrast media may be introduced to visualize soft tissues and organs.

Usually, two X-rays are taken, each at different angles (usually right angles) to obtain different views. The anteroposterior (AP), or frontal, view and a lateral view are usually taken. In an AP view of the chest the X-ray passes through the front of the chest to the back, which is pressed against the film cassette. A postero-anterior (PA) view of the chest is the opposite: the patient faces away from the X-ray beam and the chest is pressed against the film cassette. Thus, the X-ray passes through the back of the chest to the front.

Tomography

This is a special technique in which a single layer of tissue is examined. This is achieved by blurring the image of the tissues above and below the layer of tissue to be studied when the X-ray is taken.

Fluoroscopy

This is a method in which the function of organs can be directly visualized in motion on a fluorescent screen. The image inten-sifier studies this in detail. Thus, the heart beat, movement of the diaphragm, and motility of the gastrointestinal tract can be observed and recorded on videotape.

Nursing implications

The main problem with this method of investigation is that the patient is usually frightened, both by the X-ray equipment and by the possibility of a serious condition being shown on the film. It is therefore important that the nurse give the patient informa-tion about the preparation and actual procedure.

The patient is usually asked to undress to the waist (if a chest X-ray is being performed), to remove any jewellery such as necklaces, and to wear a gown. The X-ray may be performed in the X-ray department, clinic, or on the ward at the patient's bedside. The patient may be required to sit, stand, or lie on a hard, cold X-ray table, depending upon the type of film required.

However, the patient should be informed of this and also warned that it is not unusual for two or more films to be taken. The patient should be given information about the duration of the procedure (usually 10–15 minutes), sensations to be expected (cold film cassette placed against body), equipment used and staff involved (X-rays are performed by technicians called radiographers and the films are interpreted by doctors called radiologists), and probable outcome. It is important that the patient is told how and when he can find out the result of the X-ray.

It is the nurse who is usually asked by the patient about X-rays, and she should provide him with accurate information. Many patients are concerned about the amount of radiation they may be exposed to and the effects this may have. The nurse should assure the patient that, although he is receiving radiation, it is in very small amounts and is not harmful either to him or to relatives or friends. The patient will be asked if and when he has been X-rayed before, and how many times.

The '10-day rule'
In the UK, accidental irradiation of the fetus is minimized by applying the '10-day rule', which means that all women of reproductive capacity (12–50 years) will only be subjected to X-ray examination of the abdomen within the first 10 days after the start of the last menstrual cycle.

X-rays should also be avoided during the first trimester of pregnancy, because of risk of damage to the fetus.

ULTRASONOGRAPHY

Ultrasound is a relatively new non-invasive diagnostic procedure used to view body structures. An ultrasound probe called a transducer is held over the patient's body surface to direct an ultrasound beam to the tissues. The reflected sound waves or echoes from these tissues are converted to electrical impulses and recorded on an oscilloscope, moving chart recorder, or video-tape.

Ultrasound is a convenient, safe, and relatively inexpensive investigation. It is safer than radiography because it does not use ionizing radiation. Some of the structures which ultrasound examines include the brain (echoencephalography), the arteries and veins (Doppler ultrasound), the heart (echocardiography), the kidney, liver, and pelvis. It is probably best known for its use in obstetrics, where its main application is in demonstrating fetal size and growth, position of the placenta, and any obstetric problems. It is also used in amniocentesis to guide the needle through the abdominal wall. There is, at present, some degree of controversy over the use of ultrasound in obstetrics, but there is no direct evidence suggesting that it is harmful to the fetus (Stark et al., 1984).

Nursing implications

Most patients do not seem to mind undergoing this investigation. In fact, some patients are quite interested in watching the images of their heart or fetus on the oscilloscope. The actual procedure does not take long, usually 15 minutes. The procedure is performed by a technician, usually in a special department but sometimes at the bedside.

No special preparation is required, unless a pelvic or abdominal scan is being performed. For the former, a full bladder will improve visualization, and for the latter the patient should fast for 6 hours beforehand to reduce the amount of air present, which prevents viewing.

The patient is usually asked to remove clothing from the area to be scanned. He is then asked to lie supine on an examining couch. The technician applies a special lubricant to the skin surface at the site that is to be examined, and the transducer is moved by hand across the skin surface.

The purpose of the investigation should be explained in simple terms: i.e., 'to look at the size and structure of the specific organ to see if it is normal'. The procedure should be explained in sequence, and information should include the need to fast if an abdominal scan is required, or the need to drink extra amounts of fluid if a pelvic scan is required. The safety of the procedure should be stressed, and that it is not harmful either to the patient or to relatives and friends.

Once the procedure is completed, the skin is wiped dry and clean and the patient resumes his normal routine. It is important that the patient be told how and when he can find out the result of the scan.

COMPUTED TOMOGRAPHY
(COMPUTERIZED AXIAL TOMOGRAPHY)

Computed tomography (CT) scanning is an X-ray technique which uses a computer to reconstruct an image of a layer of tissue in the body. The basic components of the scanning system are the scanner, computer, and video monitor. The scanner produces a narrow X-ray beam which examines body sections from many different angles. It produces a series of cross-sectional images in sequence that build up a three-dimensional picture of the organ being studied. The CT scanner is about 100 times more sensitive than the conventional X-ray, so it detects fine structures and small changes in density. The computer calculates the amount of X-ray penetration of each tissue and displays this image in shades of grey or in colour coding, on a TV screen where it is videotaped. The information is then stored on floppy disc or magnetic tape.

The particular benefit of CT scanning is in imaging the three main cavities of the body: head, thorax, and abdomen. It is therefore performed for visualizing the size, shape, and position of the organs and other tissues in these cavities. It is mainly used for detecting cerebral lesions: i.e., haematomas, tumours, cysts, oedema, atrophy, hydrocephalus, and infarction. But it is also used on the body for detecting lesions such as tumours and cysts of the lung, liver, pancreas, and kidney.

Because these scanners are so expensive they are largely limited to large centres in the UK.

The CT scan is performed in a special department by a radiographer. The procedure takes from 45 to 90 minutes, depending on the type of scan.

The CT scanner is a large piece of equipment through which runs a short tunnel, around which the circular scanner rotates. The patient is positioned in the tunnel on a special movable trolley or table.

The procedure and its purpose are explained to the patient, who is asked to sign a consent form. The patient is requested to fast for 4 hours before scanning. If a head scan is to be performed, the patient is asked to remove any earrings, hairpins, or other ornaments. The patient is then escorted to the department and asked to lie supine on a special table with the head positioned in a cradle to keep it immobilized. The table then moves so that the head is positioned in the short tunnel in which the scanning takes place. Sometimes, a contrast medium may be indicated. The head scan takes from 45 to 60 minutes.

If an abdominal scan is to be performed, the patient will have been given instructions to follow a low-residue diet for 2 days prior to the investigation. The patient is asked to undress, remove any jewellery, and to wear a gown. He is often asked to drink a solution of contrast medium to improve visualization. The patient then lies on the table and is asked to keep still. Often he is asked to hold his breath during scanning. This scan takes about 90 minutes to perform.

Nursing implications

This is a relatively simple and painless investigation which is safe and generally non-invasive. However, many patients are under-standably apprehensive when they see the imposing equipment in the bare and clinical-looking room in which it is housed. Therefore, the nurse needs to explain carefully to the patient what is actually involved and what is required of him.

The purpose should be explained in simple terms: i.e., 'to look at the structures in the head or body to see if they are normal'. The patient should be assured that the investigation is safe and painless. The main problem is likely to be claustrophobia. Such patients can find either type of scan frightening, particularly the head scanner. Although the machine looks imposing, it is often a good idea, if practical, to accompany the patient on a short visit to the department, even if only to watch through a window.

If fasting is required the patient should be given verbal and written instructions about this and any dietary preparation he needs. Some patients are prescribed sedation, particularly if they are very anxious. The nurse should assess the need for such medication and should not be reluctant to give it if it has been prescribed. A relaxed patient is much more cooperative. He will require information about the actual procedure, staff involved, duration, sensations to be expected, and probable outcome. During the procedure, it is important that the patient appreciate the need to keep still, and possibly not to talk. He should also be informed of the sensations and noises he is likely to experience: i.e., the 'clicking' noise as the scanner moves around the head, and the temporary feeling of claustrophobia and nausea, which is not uncommon. Therefore, the patient will require ample opportunity to express his fear or concern.

A major problem for the nurse is that she cannot be with the patient throughout the procedure, and communication takes place by the operator giving instructions to the patient over a microphone. This is far from ideal, and the nurse needs to utilize her entire range of social skills to allay the patient's fears.

RADIOISOTOPE SCANNING (RADIONUCLIDE IMAGING)

A radioactive isotope is an unstable isotope which decays or disintegrates, emitting radiation or energy. The energy source is therefore inside the patient and its distribution is largely determined by the compound or vehicle to which the radioisotope (often referred to as a radionuclide) is bound chemically. The radioisotope is given orally or intravenously. Different radioisotopes have different chemical and physical properties, i.e. ^{99m}Tc (technetium), ^{131}I and ^{123}I (iodine), and ^{201}Tl (thallium). They are concentrated by certain target organs, and their distribution in healthy tissue is different from that in diseased tissue.

The external detection and localization of the radioisotope disintegration is carried out using a rectilinear scanner or a scintillation (gamma) camera detector. The information is then usually displayed on a cathode ray tube and recorded on photographic or X-ray film or on paper. A uniform colour of grey distribution is considered normal, whereas darker shades which indicate hyperfunction are referred to as hot spots, and lighter shades indicate hypofunction and are referred to as cold spots. A computer is used for the acquisition, storage, and processing of the data. Radioisotope scans do not depict structural anatomy; they show the distribution of function within the target organ. The dose given is low and results in only a small amount of radiation to the patient.

Radioisotope scans are performed to detect malfunction or abnormalities of bone, lungs, brain, heart, kidneys, liver, biliary tract, endocrine glands, and the spleen. The procedure for each organ scan varies according to the mode of administration, the interval between administration and scanning, and the form of preparation. A consent form is usually required to be signed once the procedure and its purpose have been explained to the patient.

The scan is performed in the department of nuclear medicine by a technician or a physician.

Nursing implications

Most patients are more concerned about the risk of radiation than by the actual investigation. It should therefore be stressed that the radiation dose is only small and is considered harmless to the patient, family, and others.

The procedure should be carefully explained, including the equipment used (and its safety), duration, staff involved, and likely outcome. The patient should be informed that the test is not painful, unless an intravenous injection of the radioisotope (radionuclide) is given, in which case a little discomfort may be felt.

The purpose of the scan should be explained in simple terms: i.e., 'to test the function of the specific organ', and the patient should be encouraged to express his fear or concern.

The procedure should also be explained to the patient, and will differ according to the organ being scanned. In most cases there is no need to fast, and in some cases drinking water is encouraged, i.e. for a bone and renal scan. The patient should be told there may be a waiting period between the administration of the radioisotope and the scanning, and it may be advisable to bring a book to read. The patient should be asked if he wishes to pass urine before the procedure. He is also asked to remove any clothing and jewellery from the site to be scanned. He should be warned that he may be asked to change body position during the test, but apart from that he should remain still. Depending on the type of scan to be performed, the patient may be instructed by the physician to stop taking certain drugs, and the nurse should check this, as the results of the test may be affected.

Once the radioisotope has been given, the patient should be told when he should return for the scanning. The accuracy of the test will depend on the patient arriving on time. Finally, the patient needs an explanation of the scanning equipment and the fact that the scanner will be moved over the parts of the body being studied. This will be painless, but may make certain strange noises as the radiation is detected.

Because the procedure for radioisotope scanning varies,

instructions to patients should be written on a special card to ensure he complies with them.

Once the procedure is complete, the patient should be told how and when he can obtain the results of the test.

NUCLEAR MAGNETIC RESONANCE IMAGING

Nuclear magnetic resonance (NMR) imaging is a very new technique which is becoming widely used in medicine. It employs radio-frequency (RF) radiation in the presence of a magnetic field to produce anatomical sections of the human body. The image is produced from the signals emitted when certain naturally occurring elements (mainly hydrogen) in the body are caused to resonate in the magnetic field.

The advantage of this technique is that NMR imaging is non-invasive, does not use ionizing radiation, penetrates bony structures without attenuation, and appears to be without hazard, as yet—although there is some controversy about the safety of RF radiation. In contrast with CT scanning, NMR imaging can provide images in any anatomical plane.

It seems certain, therefore, that CT and NMR imaging will soon be in direct competition. Although NMR imaging techniques are not as commercially available at the moment, it seems likely that, before long, all major centres will be equipped with NMR scanners.

THERMOGRAPHY

Thermography is a technique which measures and records heat energy from the skin surface. It is non-invasive and does not cause any discomfort to the patient. Malignant lesions cause increased metabolism, resulting in increased surface temperature and vascularity (hot spots). Two methods are used: infra-red thermography and liquid crystal thermography. In the former a microprocessor is used to allow real-time display and recording. A pictorial record is made of the infra red radiation emitted. The patient is scanned in much the same way as a photograph is taken. In the latter, a heat-sensitive crystal which is on film is used. Plates with these films are placed on the skin and changes in skin temperature are reflected on a colour map.

Usually, the patient is asked to sit in a room with a constant temperature in the range of 18–20°C, for about 15 minutes.

Thermograms are mainly used to detect lesions of the breast, particularly malignant ones. It is also being used to select the optimum site for amputation of an ischaemic limb, to diagnose spinal root compression syndromes, to evaluate drug therapy, and to assess the progress of wound healing. The full value of thermography has thus yet to be realized.

Thermography is performed in special departments or in breast-screening clinics, by a technician. The duration of the procedure is about 20 minutes.

No special preparation is usually required, although immediately before the test changes in temperature should be avoided. The patient should remove any clothing or jewellery at the site to be scanned. If this is the breast, the patient usually undresses from the neck to the waist and wears a gown. The patient is seated and photographs are taken from different angles.

Nursing implications

Thermography is painless, harmless, quick, and non-invasive, and these points should be stressed. However, for the test to be successful, the patient should be informed of the importance of avoiding sudden changes in body temperature. Factors which may cause this include environmental changes, hot or cold drinks, alcohol, cigarette smoking, cosmetics (to a lesser degree), and exercise. The patient should be advised to avoid these for a minimum of 1 hour, if possible, before the test.

The procedure and its purpose should be explained to the patient, who should be given the opportunity to express any fear or concern. The purpose should be explained in simple terms: i.e., 'to see if there are any heat changes in the tissues of the breast'. The patient should be given information about the procedure in sequence, the equipment and staff involved, the duration, and any sensations, and the expected outcome.

Female patients should be asked about their menstrual cycle. They should not have a thermogram if pregnant, menstruating, or close to their period, as the vascularity of the breasts will increase at these times, affecting the results. They should be informed that different views of the breasts will be photographed and that they should not be alarmed if repeated films are required.

Understandably, female patients having their breasts scanned will be apprehensive and frightened, especially at the actual procedure and the outcome of the test. The nurse therefore should be supportive and a good listener. Both patient and partner should be told how and when to obtain the results of the investigation. Usually, these are available within two or three days. It is a good idea to instruct women who have attended for breast scanning on how to undertake self-examination of the breast for potential lumps.

If hot spots are recorded on the breast scan, additional investigations such as mammography and/or biopsy should be performed to confirm breast cancer.

BONE MARROW ASPIRATION AND BIOPSY

This investigation involves the insertion of a needle through soft tissue and bone, in order to aspirate or obtain a biopsy of bone marrow for analysis in the laboratory.

The main indication for bone marrow aspiration and biopsy is for the diagnosis of blood disorders such as leukaemia, myelomas, polycythaemia, and pernicious anaemia.

This investigation is usually performed under a local anaesthetic on the ward by a physician. The procedure takes from 10 to 15 minutes.

The procedure and its purpose should be explained to the patient, who is asked to sign a consent form. The site normally chosen is the sternum or iliac crest (in adults). If the former, the patient is asked to undress to the waist. If the latter, the patient may be asked to remove his clothes from the waist down in order to expose the hips. The patient lies supine on the hard examining table. The skin surface area to be punctured is aseptically prepared and infiltrated with local anaesthetic. If the skin surface is hairy, it may have to be shaved beforehand.

Most patients do not require sedation, but if they are unduly apprehensive it may be necessary in order to achieve their cooperation in keeping still during the procedure.

A large-bore needle with stilette is slowly advanced through the soft tissue, periosteum, and into the bone marrow. The stilette is removed and a syringe is attached to the needle and bone marrow is aspirated. If a biopsy is required, a biopsy instrument in the form of either a wider-bore needle or trephine is screwed into the bone. The instrument is withdrawn when the biopsy has been obtained.

Nursing implications

Most patients are anxious and frightened that this may be a painful procedure. A well-informed patient will be more relaxed and cooperative. Explanation should cover such factors as procedure, equipment, sensations to be expected, duration, staff involved, and probable outcome. It is important to state that some degree of pain is involved with the actual insertion of the needle, but that the local anaesthetic will minimize it. It is also important to stress that the patient must keep still throughout the procedure, otherwise the needle may accidentally puncture a vital organ.

The purpose of the investigation should be explained in simple terms to the patient and relatives: i.e., 'to obtain and examine a piece of bone-marrow tissue for analysis in the laboratory'. They should be encouraged to ask questions. The patient should be told that sedation will be prescribed by the physician, and the effects, duration, and side-effects of the drugs used (including local anaesthetic) should also be explained. He should be given the opportunity to pass urine before the test.

Once the biopsy is completed, the nurse should apply a sterile occlusive dressing to the puncture site. She should ensure that the patient is warm and comfortable and assess whether he has any discomfort that may require analgesia.

The patient will usually want to rest for a few hours, as the procedure can be distressing and tiring, and this should be encouraged. The nurse should observe the wound site for bleeding or haematoma. She should inform the patient that it is usual to experience tenderness at the puncture site for several days and that he should take mild analgesics, which are usually prescribed.

The patient will be anxious about the outcome of the procedure and should be told how and when he can obtain the test results.

LYMPHANGIOGRAPHY

This investigation involves the introduction of a radio-opaque dye into the lymphatic system (lymphatic vessels and lymph nodes) so that it can be viewed under fluoroscopy and X-ray filming.

The main indication for performing a lymphangiogram is to identify and determine the extent of malignant lymphoma (Hodgkin's disease) and metastasis of the lymph nodes.

This investigation is performed under a local anaesthetic (sometimes a general anaesthetic is preferred), usually on the ward by a physician. The procedure takes $2\frac{1}{2}$–3 hours.

The procedure and its purpose should be explained to the patient, who is then asked to sign a consent form. The patient is not usually fasted or specially prepared, unless a general anaesthetic is thought necessary.

Sedation is usually prescribed to promote relaxation. The patient is made comfortable and informed that a dye will be injected subcutaneously between several toes of each foot to stain the lymphatic vessels of the feet. Prior to this the skin is aseptically prepared and infiltrated with local anaesthetic. A needle with tubing is then inserted into a lymphatic vessel chosen by the physician from the vessels which have been initially highlighted by the subcutaneous injection of dye. Dye is slowly infused into the cannulated lymphatic vessel by a special infusion (lymphangiographic) pump. The patient is asked to remain still during the whole procedure. Fluoroscopy is often used to follow the dye through the lymphatic vessels. A series of X-ray films are then taken of the lymphatics in the leg, pelvic, abdominal, and chest areas.

Nursing implications

Most patients are worried about the injections that are given during the procedure rather than by the procedure itself. It is therefore important to inform the patient fully and exactly about what is entailed, particularly with regard to the injections. These are painful, and although the pain is reduced by the local anaesthetic, the injection of this is itself painful. However, a patient who knows exactly what to expect will usually be more relaxed and cooperative, and the sedation will contribute to this.

The patient will also need information about the actual procedure, staff, equipment, sensations to be expected, duration, and probable outcome. The purpose of the investigation should be explained in simple terms: i.e., 'to look at the lymph vessels and lymph nodes on film to see if they are normal'.

The effects, duration, and side-effects of the drugs used (sedatives and local anaesthetic) should be explained. The patient should be told that the drugs may make him feel drowsy and relaxed, and that he will be given analgesia for any pain.

The importance of keeping still should be emphasized, and this can be aided by careful positioning and ensuring that the patient is comfortable. Because the procedure is so lengthy, it is a good idea to tell the patient to bring a book to read. He should also be asked if he wishes to pass urine before the procedure starts.

Once the procedure is completed, the patient should be advised to rest in bed for at least 12 hours. He will usually find it quite tiring, and will feel relieved when it is over.

Any pain should be controlled with analgesia, and the nurse should observe the cannulation site for signs of infection or haematoma. She should also check the legs for oedema.

The dye usually remains in the lymph nodes for 6–12 months. The dye also discolours the urine and faeces for several days, and the skin may be discoloured (usually with a bluish tinge) for 24–48 hours. The patient should be warned of these effects before the procedure begins, so that he does not become alarmed.

The nurse should appreciate that, because of the nature of the test and the reason it has been requested, the patient will be eager to know the outcome. He should therefore be told how and when he can obtain the test results, which are usually available within a few days.

References and further reading

Allan, D. & Armstrong, D. (1984) Patient attitudes towards radiographic examinations involving contrast media. *Clin. Radiol.* **35**, 457–459.

Andrew, E. R. (1984) A historical review of NMR and its clinical applications. *Brit. Med. Bull.* **40**, 2, 115–119.

Husband, J. E. & Fry, I. K. (1981) *Computed Tomography of the Body.* London: Macmillan.

Kreel, L. *Ed.* (1979) *Medical Imaging: a Basic Course.* Aylesbury: HM & M.

Maisey, M. N., Britton, K. E. & Gilday, D. L. *Ed.* (1983) *Clinical Nuclear Medicine.* London: Chapman & Hall.

Russell, J. G. B. (1984) How dangerous are diagnostic X-rays? *Clin. Radiol.* **35**, 347–351.

Stark, C. R., Orleans, M., Haverkamp, A. D. & Murphy, J. (1984)
Short- and long-term risks after exposure to diagnostic ultrasound in
utero. *Obstet. Gynecol.* **63**, 2, 194–200.
Walker, S. (1983) Understanding X-ray films. *J. Emerg. Nurs.* **9**,
315–323.
Wilson-Barnett, J. (1978) Patients' emotional responses to barium X-
rays. *J. Adv. Nurs.* 3, 37–48.

Index